2024 Ultimate

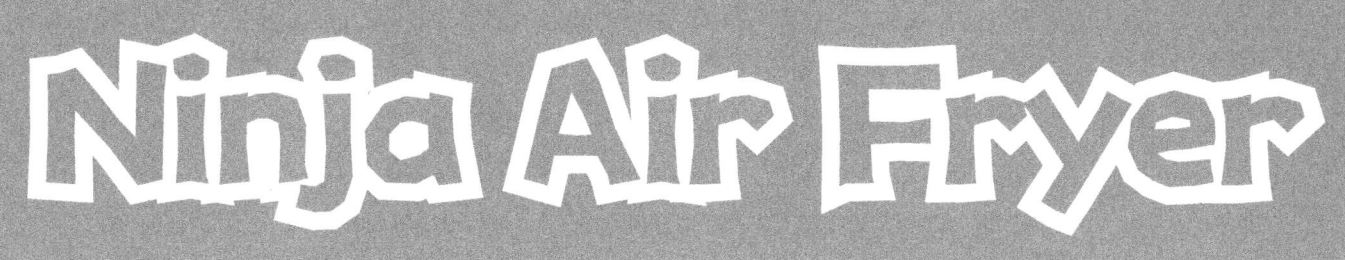

Cookbook

1800 | Days of Easy & Flavourful Ninja Air Fryer Recipes for Beginners With Step-by-Step Instructions | Breakfast, Lunch, Dinner, Snacks & More | UK Measurements

Lola O'Donnell

All Rights Reserved.

The content contained within this book may not be reproduced, duplicated, or transmitted without direct written permission from the author or the publisher. Under no circumstances will any blame or legal responsibility be held against the publisher, or author, for any damages, reparation, or monetary loss due to the information contained within this book, either directly or indirectly.

Legal Notice:

This book is copyright protected. It is only for personal use. You cannot amend, distribute, sell, use, quote or paraphrase any part, or the content within this book, without the consent of the author or publisher.

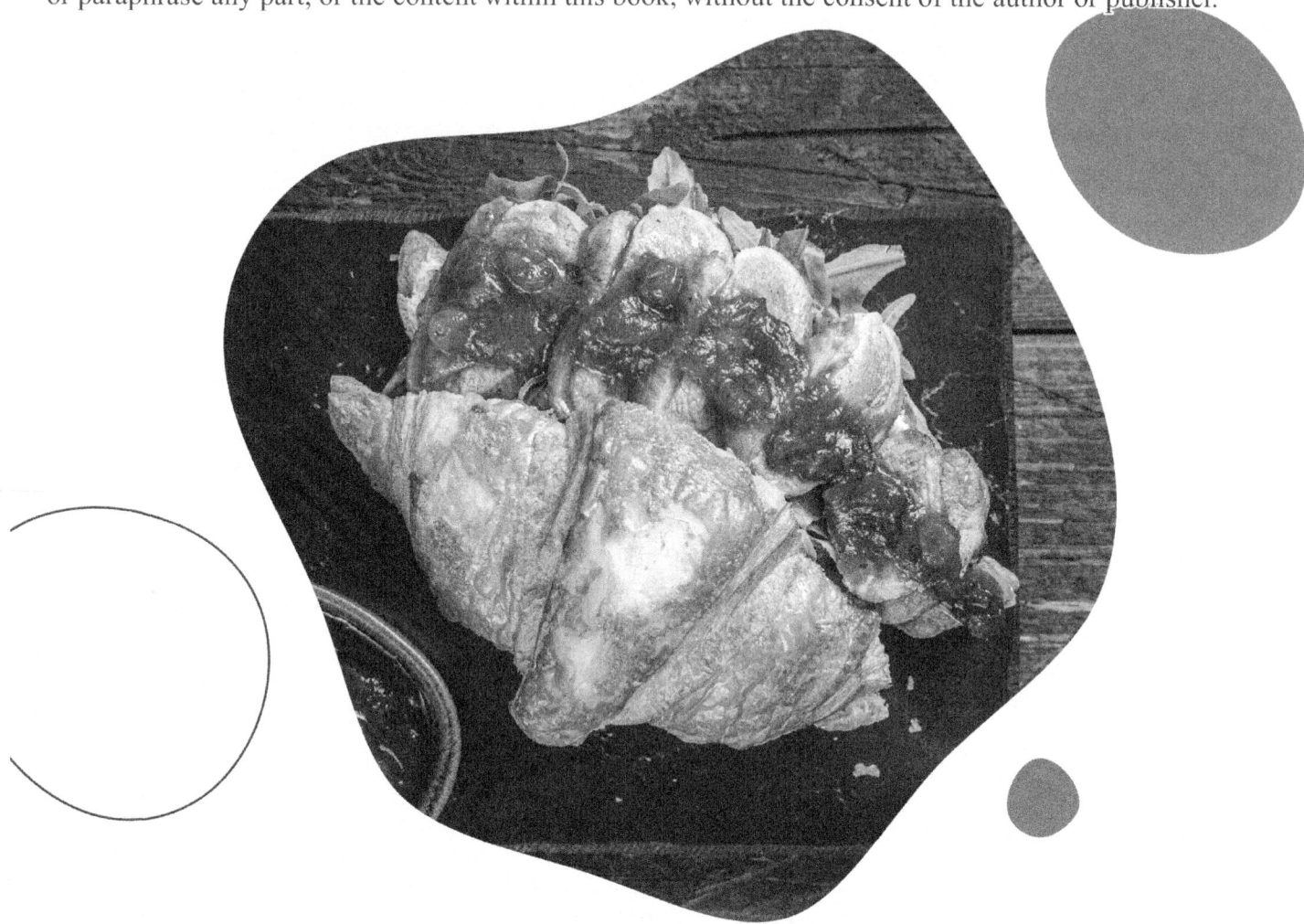

Disclaimer Notice:

Please note the information contained within this document is for educational and entertainment purposes only. All effort has been executed to present accurate, up to date, reliable, complete information. No warranties of any kind are declared or implied. Readers acknowledge that the author is not engaged in the rendering of legal, financial, medical, or professional advice. The content within this book has been derived from various sources. Please consult a licensed professional before attempting any techniques outlined in this book. By reading this document, the reader agrees that under no circumstances is the author responsible for any losses, direct or indirect, that are incurred as a result of the use of the information contained within this document, including, but not limited to, errors, omissions, or inaccuracies.

CONTENTS

INTRODUCTION 7

How does an Air Fryer work?.................................8
Is Cooking With an Air Fryer Healthy? 8
Who is an Air Fryer suitable for?............................8
Tips for successful cooking with an Air Fryer 9

Bread And Breakfast.................... 11

Lemon Monkey Bread 12
Favorite Blueberry Muffins....................................12
Baked Eggs With Bacon-tomato Sauce 13
Breakfast Chimichangas 13
Easy Caprese Flatbread 14
Meaty Omelet..14
Ham & Cheese Sandwiches 14
Egg & Bacon Pockets 15
Buttermilk Biscuits 15
Mascarpone Iced Cinnamon Rolls 16
Eggless Mung Bean Tart 16
Canadian Bacon & Cheese Sandwich 17
Herby Parmesan Pita 17
Cheddar & Egg Scramble 17
Effortless Toffee Zucchini Bread 18
Ham And Cheddar Gritters 18
All-in-one Breakfast Toast 19
Crustless Broccoli, Roasted Pepper, And Fontina

Quiche...19
Huevos Rancheros 20
Egg And Sausage Crescent Rolls 20
American Biscuits 21
Healthy Granola 21

Appetizers And Snacks 22

Corn Dog Bites 23
Indian Cauliflower Tikka Bites 23
Cholula Avocado Fries 24
Chicken Shawarma Bites 24
Asian Five-spice Wings 24
Chinese-style Potstickers 25
Beet Chips 25
Cocktail Beef Bites 25
Classic Potato Chips 26
Buffalo Bites 26
Black-olive Poppers 26
Cauliflower "tater" Tots 27
Buffalo Wings 27
Charred Shishito Peppers......................................28
Cheddar Stuffed Pepper 28
Artichoke Samosas..28
Baba Ghanouj..29
Hot Garlic Kale Chips...29
Cayenne-spiced Roasted Pecans 30

Individual Pizzas 30

Vegetarian & Vegan Recipes 31

Roast Cauliflower & Broccoli 32

Potato Gratin 32

Sweet Potato Taquitos 32

Cheese, Tomato & Pesto Crustless Quiches 33

Butternut Squash Fries 33

Bbq Soy Curls 33

Spicy Spanish Potatoes 33

Orange Zingy Cauliflower 34

Mini Quiche 34

Bagel Pizza 34

Ratatouille 35

Courgette Meatballs 35

Paneer Tikka 35

Vegan Fried Ravioli 36

Camembert & Soldiers 36

Aubergine Parmigiana 36

Spinach And Egg Air Fryer Breakfast Muffins 37

Veggie Bakes 37

Parmesan Truffle Oil Fries 37

Broccoli Cheese 37

Artichoke Pasta 38

Crispy Potato Peels 38

Tomato And Herb Tofu 38

Sandwiches And Burgers Recipes.. 39

Inside Out Cheeseburgers 40

Mexican Cheeseburgers 40

Provolone Stuffed Meatballs 41

Black Bean Veggie Burgers 41

Inside-out Cheeseburgers 42

Salmon Burgers 42

Dijon Thyme Burgers 43

Chicken Apple Brie Melt 43

Turkey Burgers 44

Perfect Burgers 44

Chicken Spiedies 45

Sausage And Pepper Subs 45

White Bean Veggie Burgers 46

Chicken Saltimbocca Sandwiches 46

Chicken Gyros 47

Eggplant Parmesan Subs 47

Reuben Sandwiches 48

Chili Cheese Dogs 48

Best-ever Roast Beef Sandwiches 49

Asian Glazed Meatballs 49

Fish And Seafood Recipes 50

Pecan-orange Crusted Striped Bass 51

Maple-crusted Salmon 51

Cajun Flounder Fillets 52

Lime Bay Scallops 52

Caribbean Skewers 52

Beer-breaded Halibut Fish Tacos 53

Feta & Shrimp Pita 53

Buttered Swordfish Steaks 54

Lemon & Herb Crusted Salmon 54

Garlic And Dill Salmon 54

Basil Crab Cakes With Fresh Salad 55
Mahi-mahi "burrito" Fillets 55
Basil Mushroom & Shrimp Spaghetti 56
Malaysian Shrimp With Sambal Mayo 56
Dilly Red Snapper 57
Halibut With Coleslaw 57
Bbq Fried Oysters 57
Coconut Jerk Shrimp 58
Mahi Mahi With Cilantro-chili Butter 58
Herb-rubbed Salmon With Avocado 59
Black Cod With Grapes, Fennel, Pecans, And Kale 59
Californian Tilapia 60
Lime Flaming Halibut 60
Hot Calamari Rings 60

Vegetable Side Dishes Recipes.. 61

Roasted Brussels Sprouts With Bacon 62
Asiago Broccoli 62
Balsamic Beet Chips 62
Hush Puppies 63
Mashed Sweet Potato Tots 63
Honey-roasted Parsnips 64
Cheese Sage Cauliflower 64
Za'atar Bell Peppers 64
Tuna Platter 65
Buttery Stuffed Tomatoes 65
Fried Eggplant Balls 66
Five-spice Roasted Sweet Potatoes 66
Butternut Medallions With Honey Butter And Sage.. 67

Greek-inspired Ratatouille 67
Moroccan Cauliflower 68
Speedy Baked Caprese With Avocado 68
Street Corn 68
Gorgonzola Stuffed Mushrooms 69
Caraway Seed Pretzel Sticks 69
Almond-crusted Zucchini Fries 69
Baked Shishito Peppers 70
Fried Eggplant Slices 70
Corn On The Cob 70
Stuffed Onions 71
Turkish Mutabal (eggplant Dip) 71

Beef, pork & Lamb Recipes 72

Blackberry Bbq Glazed Country-style Ribs 73
Citrus Pork Lettuce Wraps 73
Glazed Meatloaf 74
Balsamic London Broil 74
Crispy Pork Escalopes 75
Berbere Beef Steaks 75
Boneless Ribeye Steaks 75
Cinnamon-stick Kofta Skewers 76
Asian-style Flank Steak 76
Balsamic Marinated Rib Eye Steak With Balsamic Fried Cipollini Onions 77
Egg Stuffed Pork Meatballs 77
Carne Asada Recipes 78
Beef Brazilian Empanadas 78
Homemade Pork Gyoza 79
Carne Asada 79

Cajun Pork Loin Chops 80
Chipotle Pork Meatballs 80
Garlic-buttered Rib Eye Steak 80
French-style Steak Salad 81
Cal-mex Chimichangas 81

Poultry Recipes 82

Harissa Chicken Wings 83
Chicken Strips 83
Garlic Chicken 83
Granny Pesto Chicken Caprese 84
Farmer's Fried Chicken 84
Chicken Chunks 85
Crunchy Chicken Strips 85
Buttery Chicken Legs 85
Coconut Chicken With Apricot-ginger Sauce 86
Chicken Flautas 86
Chicken Cordon Bleu 87
Irresistible Cheesy Chicken Sticks 87
Chicago-style Turkey Meatballs 88
Cajun Fried Chicken 88
Gruyère Asparagus & Chicken Quiche 88
Cal-mex Turkey Patties 89
Creole Chicken Drumettes 89
Chicken Flatbread Pizza With Spinach 89
Chicken Cordon Bleu Patties 90
Crispy Chicken Parmesan 90

Desserts And Sweets 91

Caramel Apple Crumble 92

Mango-chocolate Custard 92
Chewy Coconut Cake 93
Mixed Berry Pie 93
Molten Chocolate Almond Cakes 94
Honey-roasted Mixed Nuts 94
Baked Apple 95
Cinnamon Canned Biscuit Donuts 95
Fast Brownies 95
Black And Blue Clafoutis 96
Glazed Cherry Turnovers 96
Apple Dumplings 97
Annie's Chocolate Chunk Hazelnut Cookies 97
Fried Twinkies 98
Coconut Macaroons 98
Carrot-oat Cake Muffins 98
Mixed Berry Hand Pies 99
Chocolate Macaroons 99

Measurement Conversions 100

How to Reduce Food Waste 102

Appendix : Recipes Index 104

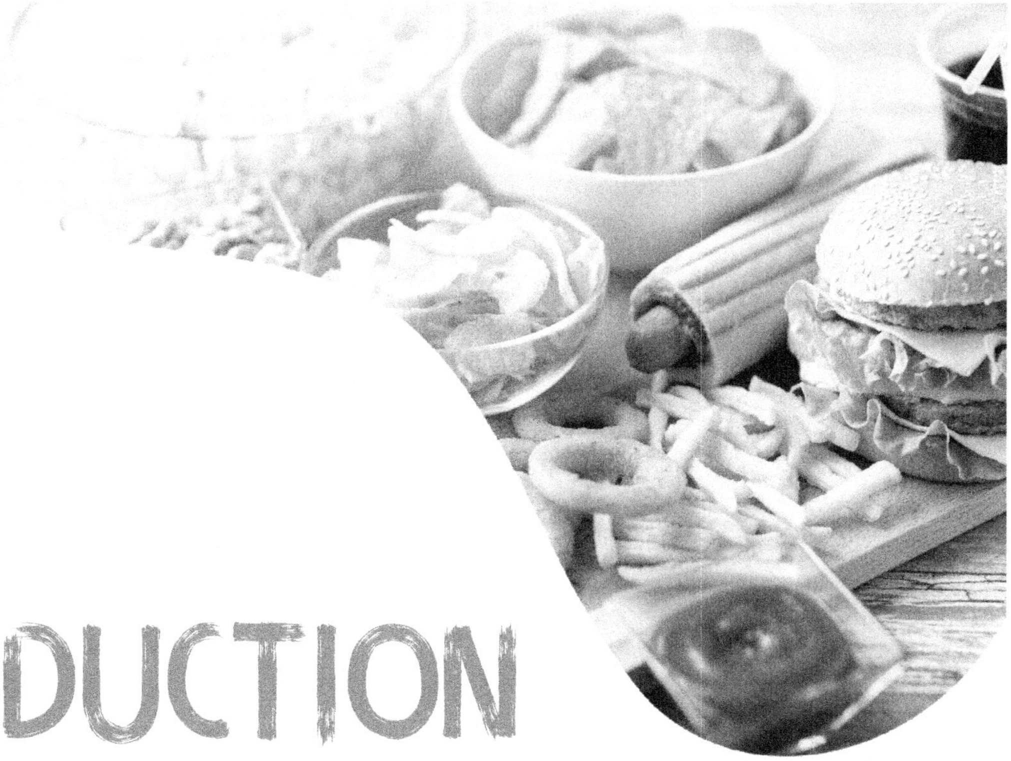

INTRODUCTION

Lola O'Donnell is a culinary enthusiast with a passion for creating delicious and healthy meals. With a background in nutrition and a career as a registered dietitian, Lola has always been dedicated to promoting balanced and wholesome eating habits. Her journey towards writing the "Ninja Air Fryer Cookbook" was born out of a desire to make cooking enjoyable and health-conscious for everyone.

Drawing upon her years of experience in the field of nutrition and her love for culinary exploration, Lola embarked on the process of crafting this cookbook. Her goal was to harness the incredible potential of the Ninja Air Fryer, a kitchen appliance renowned for its versatility and ability to cook with less oil, without sacrificing flavor. The cookbook was meticulously crafted to provide readers with a diverse selection of recipes, each thoughtfully designed to be easy to follow, nutritious, and, most importantly, delicious.

Lola's approach to writing the "Ninja Air Fryer Cookbook" was rooted in her dedication to promoting healthy eating without compromising on taste. With her expertise in nutrition, she ensured that each recipe not only catered to the palate but also aligned with dietary guidelines, making it a valuable resource for those seeking to make mindful food choices.

As an author, Lola's mission is clear—to empower individuals of all culinary backgrounds to embrace the art of air frying. Through her cookbook, she invites readers to explore the world of crispy, flavorful dishes while maintaining a health-conscious approach to cooking. Lola's passion for food, coupled with her professional expertise, shines through in every recipe, making the "Ninja Air Fryer Cookbook" a trusted companion for those looking to savor the joy of cooking and eating well.

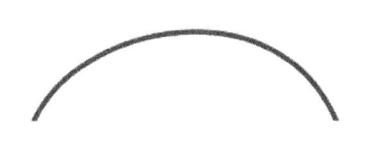

HOW DOES AN AIR FRYER WORK?

An air fryer is one of the most popular kitchen appliances out there. It's essentially a compact portable convection oven, which sits on your countertop and uses heat to bake. To clarify, despite the name, it does not fry and is not comparable to a deep fryer — it uses much less oil. This definitely makes it the healthier option of the two.

Each air fryer contains a heating element as well as a small fan which distributes the hot air across the space. These appliances are renowned for producing crispy and tender results quickly, with convenience at the core of the design. Depending on the type of air fryer you choose, they can also be used to bake, roast and broil as well, which opens up a wide range of recipe ideas.

IS COOKING WITH AN AIR FRYER HEALTHY?

The air fryer's big appeal is that it creates a very crispy texture with minimal oil, making it a healthy alternative to traditional deep frying. With an air fryer, simply tossing ingredients in a few teaspoons of oil (or skipping the oil altogether with some recipes) results in a delectably crunchy dish but with significantly less fat and calories.

WHO IS AN AIR FRYER SUITABLE FOR?

Busy Individuals: Air fryers are perfect for people with hectic schedules who want to prepare quick and convenient meals. They significantly reduce cooking times and require minimal supervision, making meal preparation efficient.

Health-Conscious Eaters: For those looking to reduce their oil intake and opt for healthier cooking methods, air fryers are an excellent choice. They allow you to enjoy crispy and delicious food with significantly less oil compared to traditional frying.

Weight Watchers: If you're on a weight management journey, an air fryer can help you enjoy your favorite fried foods with fewer calories. It's a great way to indulge in crispy snacks and dishes without compromising your dietary goals.

Families: Air fryers are family-friendly appliances, capable of preparing large batches of food quickly. They're perfect for busy parents who want to cook meals for their family without spending excessive time in the kitchen.

Cooking Enthusiasts: Even seasoned cooks can appreciate the versatility of an air fryer. It allows for creative experimentation with a wide range of recipes, from appetizers to desserts.

Small Kitchen Owners: Air fryers are compact and take up minimal counter space, making them ideal for individuals with limited kitchen space or those who live in smaller apartments.

Elderly Individuals: Air fryers are user-friendly and require minimal manual effort. This makes them suitable for older adults who may prefer easy-to-use appliances for meal preparation.

Air Fryer Cookbook

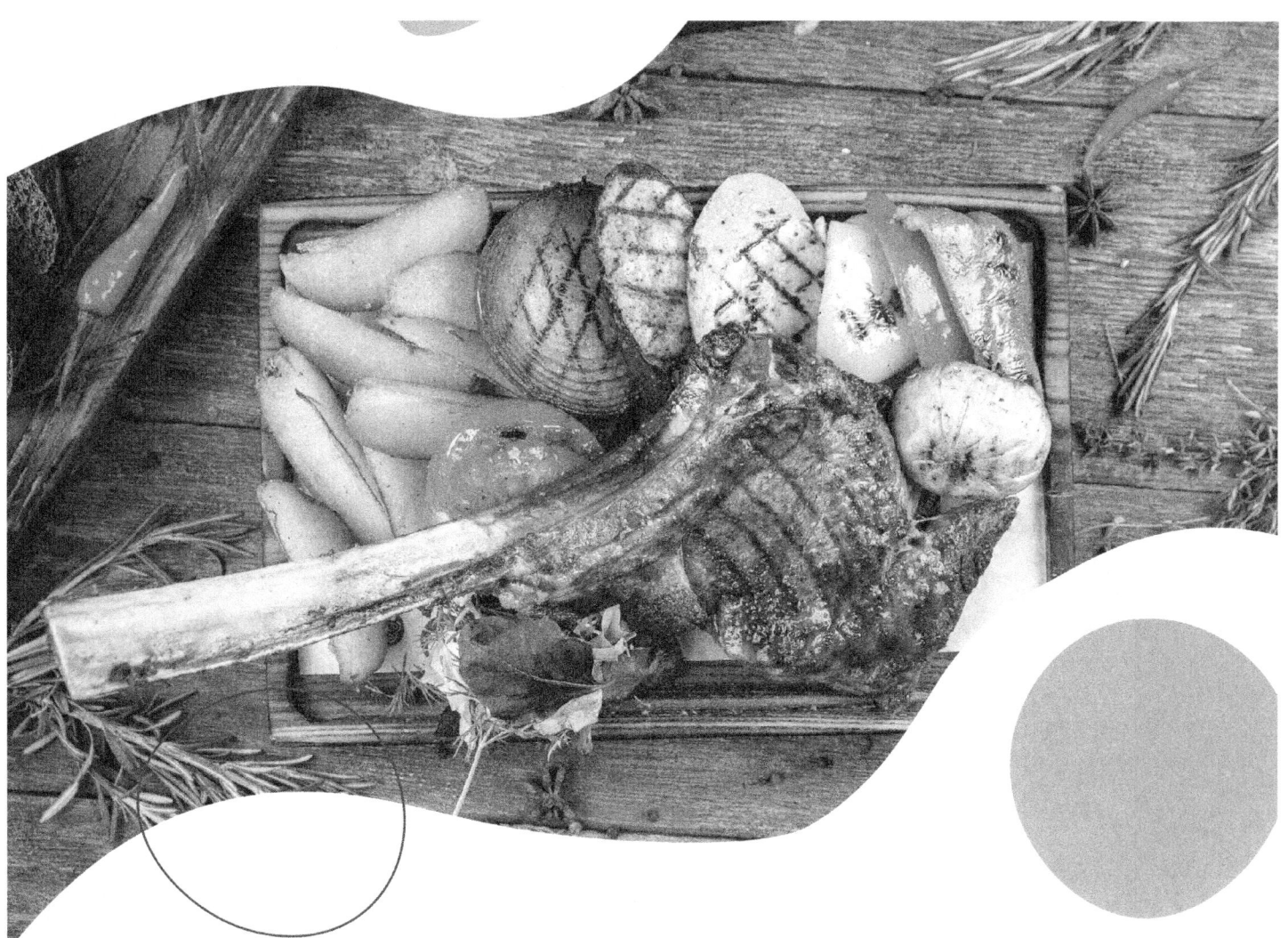

Anyone Seeking Convenience: Ultimately, air fryers are suitable for anyone who values convenience in the kitchen. Whether you're a novice cook or an experienced chef, the simplicity and speed of air frying can make meal preparation easier and more enjoyable.

TIPS FOR SUCCESSFUL COOKING WITH AN AIR FRYER

PREHEAT THE AIR FRYER

Just like with a conventional oven, it's a good practice to preheat your air fryer. Preheating helps ensure even cooking and consistent results.

USE THE RIGHT TEMPERATURE

Follow the recommended temperature settings in your air fryer recipe. Most air fryers have adjustable temperature controls, so you can customize the cooking temperature for different dishes.

DON'T OVERCROWD THE BASKET

To allow for proper air circulation and even cooking, avoid overcrowding the air fryer basket. Cook food in batches if necessary.

USE A LITTLE OIL

While air frying requires less oil than traditional frying, some recipes may benefit from a light coating of oil on the food. Use a cooking spray or a brush to apply a small amount of oil to enhance crispiness.

SHAKE OR FLIP THE FOOD

For even cooking and consistent browning, shake or flip the food in the basket halfway through the cooking time. This helps ensure that all sides are evenly exposed to the circulating hot air.

USE PARCHMENT PAPER OR LINERS

To make cleanup easier and prevent food from sticking to the basket, consider using parchment paper or specially designed air fryer liners. Be sure to use liners that are safe for air frying.

MIND THE SIZE OF FOOD

Cut food items into similar-sized pieces to ensure uniform cooking. Smaller pieces may cook faster, so keep an eye on them to avoid overcooking.

EXPERIMENT AND ADJUST

Air frying may require some trial and error to get your preferred results. Don't be afraid to experiment with different cooking times and temperatures to find the perfect settings for your favorite dishes.

CLEAN REGULARLY

Proper maintenance is essential for the longevity of your air fryer. Clean the basket, tray, and any removable parts after each use according to the manufacturer's instructions.

ADAPT RECIPES

You can adapt many of your favorite fried recipes for air frying. Experiment with different coatings, seasonings, and cooking times to achieve the desired taste and texture.

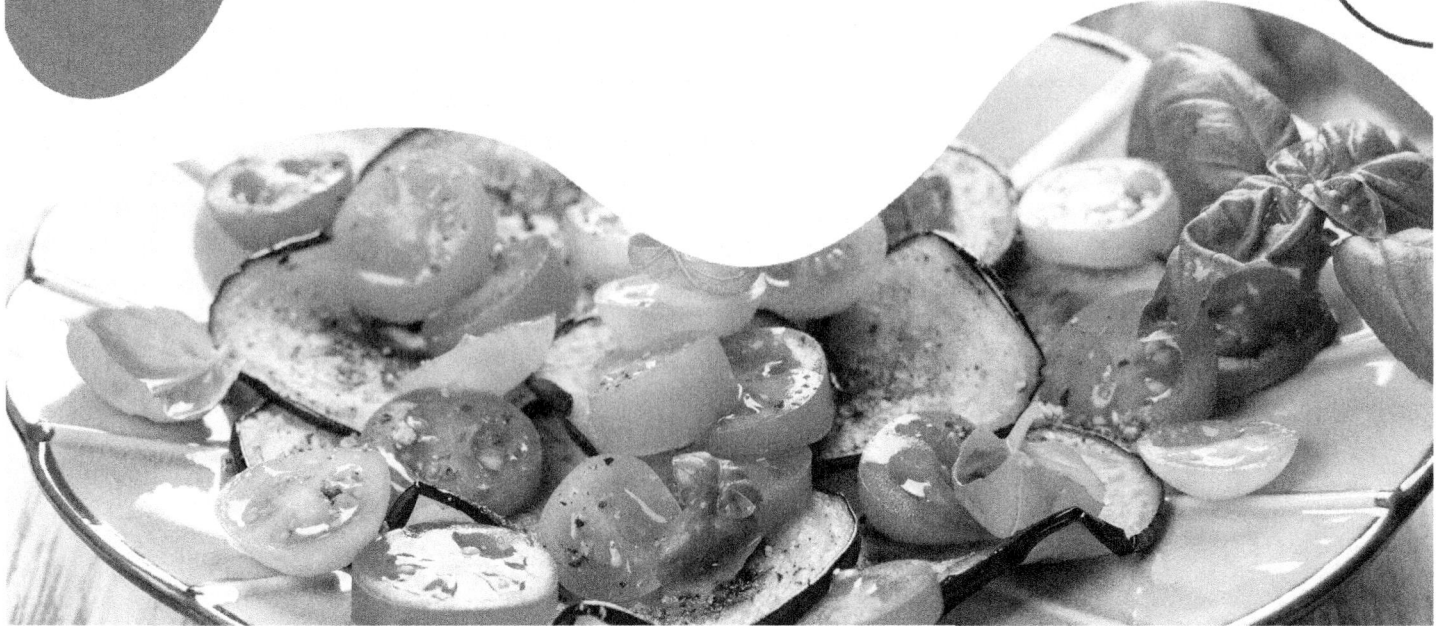

Bread And Breakfast

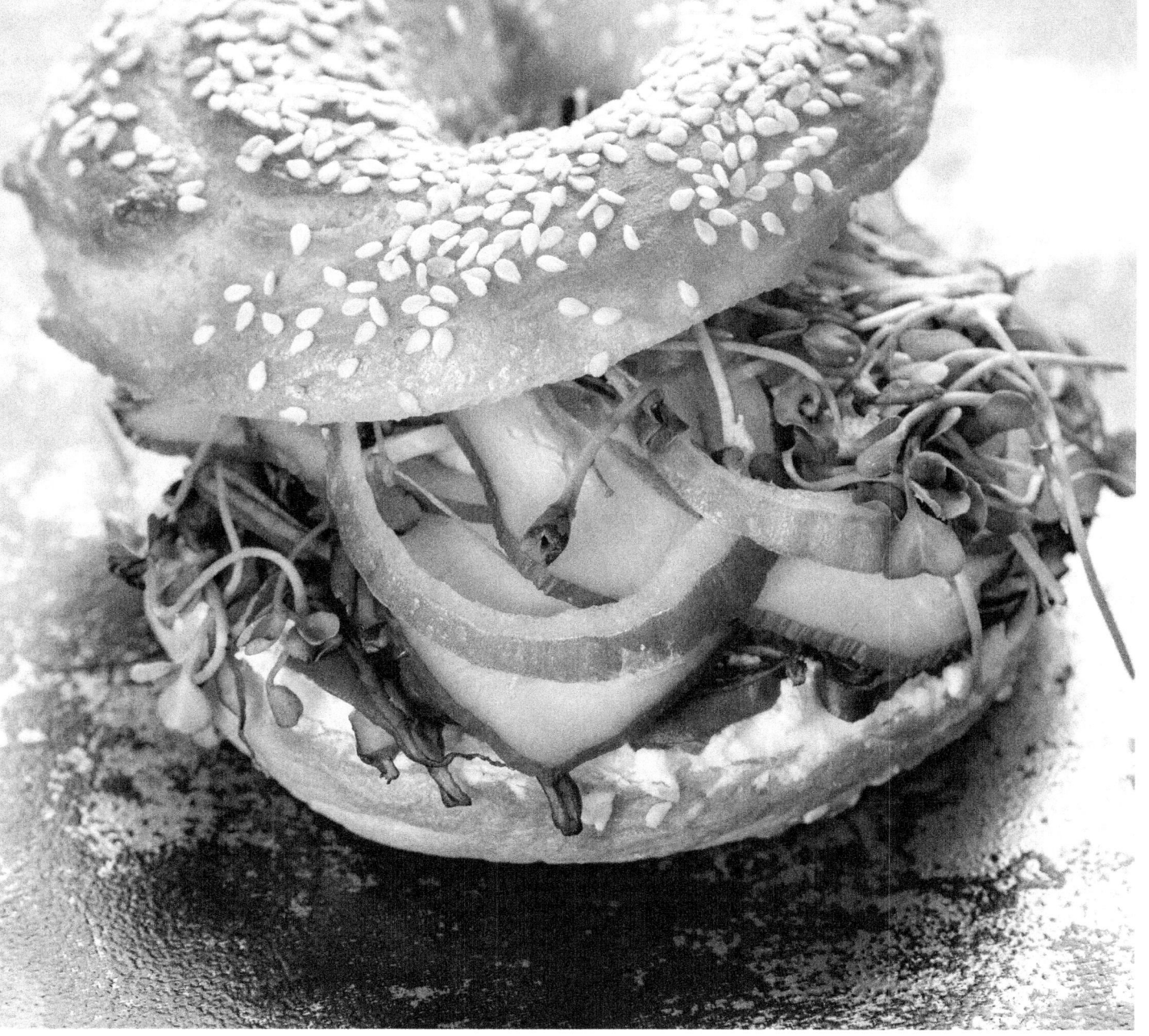

Bread And Breakfast

Lemon Monkey Bread

Servings: 4

Cooking Time: 15 Minutes

Ingredients:

- 1 can refrigerated biscuits
- ¼ cup white sugar
- 3 tbsp brown sugar
- ½ tsp ground cinnamon
- 1 lemon, zested
- ¼ tsp ground nutmeg
- 3 tbsp melted butter

Directions:

1. Preheat your air fryer to 350°F (175°C).
2. Open the can of refrigerated biscuits and separate them into individual biscuits.
3. Cut each biscuit into 4 equal pieces.
4. In a bowl, mix together the white sugar, brown sugar, lemon zest, ground cinnamon, and ground nutmeg. This will be your coating for the biscuit pieces.
5. Have the melted butter ready in a separate bowl.
6. Dip each biscuit piece into the melted butter, ensuring it's coated on all sides.
7. Roll the buttered biscuit piece in the cinnamon sugar mixture until it's well coated.
8. Place the coated biscuit pieces in a baking pan, arranging them evenly.
9. Once your air fryer is preheated, place the baking pan with the biscuit pieces into the air fryer.
10. Air-fry the lemon monkey bread at 350°F for 6-9 minutes or until they are golden brown and cooked through.
11. Carefully remove the pan from the air fryer (it will be hot) and let the monkey bread cool for about 5 minutes before serving, as the sugar coating will be very hot.
12. Serve and enjoy your delicious Lemon Monkey Bread!

Favorite Blueberry Muffins

Servings: 8

Cooking Time: 25 Minutes

Ingredients:

- 125 grams all-purpose flour
- 2.5 ml baking soda
- 80 grams granulated sugar
- 1.25 ml salt
- 15 ml lemon juice
- 5 ml lemon zest
- 60 ml milk
- 2.5 ml vanilla extract
- 1 egg
- 15 ml vegetable oil
- 60 grams halved blueberries
- 15 ml powdered sugar

Directions:

1. Preheat the air fryer to 190°C (375°F).
2. In a bowl, combine the dry ingredients: all-purpose flour, baking soda, granulated sugar, and salt.
3. Mix 60 ml of fresh milk with 5 ml of lemon juice and leave it for 10 minutes to create buttermilk.
4. In another bowl, mix together the buttermilk, lemon zest, vanilla extract, egg, and vegetable oil.
5. Pour the wet ingredients into the bowl of dry ingredients and gently toss to combine.
6. Fold in the halved blueberries into the muffin batter.
7. Spoon the muffin mixture into 8 greased silicone cupcake liners.
8. Place the muffin liners in the air fryer and bake for 6-8 minutes or until the muffins are cooked through and golden.
9. Allow the muffins to cool on a cooling rack.
10. Serve the muffins sprinkled with powdered sugar.

Baked Eggs With Bacon-tomato Sauce

Servings: 1

Cooking Time: 12 Minutes

Ingredients:

- 5ml olive oil
- 10g finely chopped onion
- 1g chopped fresh oregano
- A pinch of crushed red pepper flakes
- 400g (14-ounce) can crushed or diced tomatoes
- Salt and freshly ground black pepper
- 2 slices of bacon, chopped
- 2 large eggs
- 25g grated Cheddar cheese
- Fresh parsley, chopped

Directions:

1. Begin by making the tomato sauce. Preheat a medium saucepan over medium heat on the stovetop. Add the olive oil and sauté the onion, oregano, and pepper flakes for 5 minutes. Add the canned tomatoes and bring them to a simmer. Season with salt and freshly ground black pepper, then simmer for 10 minutes.
2. Meanwhile, preheat your air fryer to 200°C (400°F) and pour a small amount of water into the bottom of the air fryer drawer to prevent any grease drips from burning and smoking.
3. Place the chopped bacon in the air fryer basket and air-fry at 200°C (400°F) for 5 minutes, shaking the basket occasionally.
4. When the bacon is almost crispy, remove it and place it on a paper towel-lined plate. Rinse out the air fryer drawer to remove the bacon grease.
5. Transfer the tomato sauce to a shallow 7-inch pie dish. Crack the eggs on top of the sauce and scatter the cooked bacon back on top. Season with salt and freshly ground black pepper.
6. Using an aluminum foil sling (fold a long piece of aluminum foil in half lengthwise twice to create a roughly 66cm by 7.6cm strip), place it under the pie dish. Hold the ends of the foil to move the pie dish in and out of the air fryer basket. Tuck the ends of the foil beside the pie dish while it cooks in the air fryer.
7. Air-fry at 200°C (400°F) for 5 minutes, or until the eggs are cooked to your liking.
8. Sprinkle the grated Cheddar cheese on top and air-fry for an additional 2 minutes until the cheese has melted.
9. Remove the pie dish from the air fryer, sprinkle with chopped parsley, and allow the eggs to cool for a few minutes.
10. Serve your delightful Baked Eggs with Bacon-Tomato Sauce, and enjoy with some toasted buttered bread from your air fryer!

Breakfast Chimichangas

Servings: 4

Cooking Time: 8 Minutes

Ingredients:

- Four 8-inch flour tortillas
- 120ml canned refried beans
- 240ml scrambled eggs
- 120ml grated cheddar or Monterey jack cheese
- 15ml vegetable oil
- 240ml salsa

Directions:

1. Lay the flour tortillas out flat on a cutting board.
2. In the center of each tortilla, spread 30ml (2 tablespoons) of refried beans.
3. Next, add 60ml (1/4 cup) of scrambled eggs and 30ml (2 tablespoons) of cheese to each tortilla.
4. To fold the tortillas, begin on the left side and fold to the center. Then, fold the right side into the center. Next, fold the bottom and top down and roll over to completely seal the chimichanga.
5. Using a pastry brush or oil mister, brush the tops of the tortilla packages with oil.
6. Preheat your air fryer to 200°C (400°F) for 4 minutes.
7. Place the chimichangas into the air fryer basket, seam side down, and air fry for 4 minutes.
8. Using tongs, turn over the chimichangas and cook for an additional 2 to 3 minutes or until they are light golden brown.
9. Serve your delicious Breakfast Chimichangas with salsa.
10. Enjoy your meal!

Easy Caprese Flatbread

Servings: 2

Cooking Time: 15 Minutes

Ingredients:

- 1 fresh mozzarella ball, sliced
- 1 flatbread
- 2 tsp olive oil
- 1/4 garlic clove, minced
- 1 egg
- 1/8 tsp salt
- 30 grams diced tomato
- 6 basil leaves
- 1/2 tsp dried oregano
- 1/2 tsp balsamic vinegar

Directions:

1. Preheat the air fryer to 190°C (380°F).
2. Lightly brush the top of the flatbread with olive oil, then sprinkle minced garlic evenly over it.
3. Crack the egg into a small bowl and sprinkle it with salt.
4. Place the flatbread into the air fryer basket and gently pour the egg onto the top of the flatbread.
5. Top the flatbread with diced tomatoes, mozzarella slices, dried oregano, and basil leaves.
6. Air-fry for 6 minutes until the flatbread becomes crispy and the toppings are cooked.
7. When ready, remove the Caprese flatbread from the air fryer and drizzle it with balsamic vinegar.
8. Let it cool for 5 minutes, then slice and serve.

Meaty Omelet

Servings: 4

Cooking Time: 20 Minutes

Ingredients:

- 6 eggs
- ½ cup grated Swiss cheese
- 3 breakfast sausages, sliced
- 8 bacon strips, sliced
- Salt and pepper to taste

Directions:

1. Preheat your air fryer to 360°F (182°C).
2. In a bowl, crack the eggs and beat them.
3. Stir in the grated Swiss cheese, sliced breakfast sausages, and sliced bacon into the beaten eggs.
4. Grease or use a suitable non-stick air fryer-safe baking dish or pan. You can also line it with parchment paper for easier cleanup.
5. Pour the egg mixture into the greased or lined baking dish.
6. Place the baking dish with the egg mixture into the preheated air fryer.
7. Bake the omelet in the air fryer at 360°F for approximately 15 minutes or until the top is golden brown and the omelet is cooked through.
8. Carefully remove the omelet from the air fryer.
9. Season the omelet with salt and pepper to taste.
10. Slice the omelet into wedges or squares, and it's ready to be served.

Ham & Cheese Sandwiches

Servings: 2

Cooking Time: 15 Minutes

Ingredients:

- 1 tsp butter
- 4 slices of bread
- 4 slices of deli ham
- 4 slices of Cheddar cheese
- 4 thick tomato slices
- 1 tsp dried oregano

Directions:

1. Preheat the air fryer to 190°C (370°F).
2. Spread ½ tsp of butter on one side of each slice of bread and sprinkle with dried oregano.
3. On one of the slices, layer 2 slices of ham, 2 slices of Cheddar cheese, and 2 slices of tomato on the unbuttered side.
4. Place another slice of bread, unbuttered side down, onto the toppings to create a sandwich.
5. Place the sandwiches with the buttered side down into the air fryer basket.
6. Bake for 8 minutes, flipping the sandwiches once during cooking, until they are crispy and golden.
7. Let the sandwiches cool slightly, cut them in half, and serve.

Egg & Bacon Pockets

Servings: 4

Cooking Time: 50 Minutes

Ingredients:

- 30 ml olive oil
- 4 bacon slices, chopped
- 1/4 red bell pepper, diced
- 80 ml scallions, chopped
- 4 eggs, beaten
- 80 ml grated Swiss cheese
- 125 grams flour
- 7.5 grams baking powder
- 2.5 grams salt
- 240 ml Greek yogurt
- 1 egg white, beaten
- 10 ml Italian seasoning
- 15 ml Tabasco sauce

Directions:

1. Warm the olive oil in a skillet over medium heat and add the chopped bacon. Stir-fry for 3-4 minutes or until it becomes crispy.
2. Add the diced red bell pepper and chopped scallions to the skillet and sauté for another 3-4 minutes.
3. Pour in the beaten eggs and stir-fry to scramble them for about 3 minutes. Stir in the grated Swiss cheese and set aside to cool.
4. Sift the flour, baking powder, and salt into a bowl. Add the Greek yogurt and mix together until well combined.
5. Transfer the dough to a floured workspace and knead it for 3 minutes or until it becomes smooth.
6. Divide the dough into 4 equal balls and roll out each ball into a round disc.
7. Divide the bacon-egg mixture equally between the rounds.
8. Fold the dough over the filling and seal the edges with a fork.
9. Brush the pockets with beaten egg white and sprinkle them with Italian seasoning.
10. Preheat the air fryer to 180°C (350°F).
11. Arrange the pockets on the greased frying basket in a single layer.
12. Bake for 9-11 minutes, flipping them once, until they turn golden.
13. Serve your Egg & Bacon Pockets with Tabasco sauce.

Buttermilk Biscuits

Servings: 4

Cooking Time: 9 Minutes

Ingredients:

- 120g plain flour
- 1½ teaspoons baking powder
- ¼ teaspoon baking soda
- ¼ teaspoon salt
- 56g butter, cut into tiny cubes
- 60ml buttermilk, plus 30ml (2 tablespoons)
- Cooking spray

Directions:

1. Preheat the air fryer to 165°C (330°F).
2. In a medium-sized bowl, combine the plain flour, baking powder, baking soda, and salt. Stir together.
3. Add the cubed butter to the dry ingredients and cut it into the flour using knives or a pastry blender until the mixture resembles breadcrumbs.
4. Pour in 60ml of buttermilk and stir it into the mixture until you have a stiff dough.
5. Divide the dough into 4 equal portions and shape each portion into a large biscuit. If the dough is too sticky to handle, you can stir in 1 or 2 more tablespoons of flour to make it firmer.
6. Spray the air fryer basket with nonstick cooking spray to prevent sticking.
7. Place the biscuits in the basket and cook at 165°C (330°F) for 9 minutes.

Mascarpone Iced Cinnamon Rolls

Servings: 6

Cooking Time: 40 Minutes

Ingredients:

- For the Cinnamon Rolls:
- ¼ cup mascarpone cheese, softened
- 9 oz puff pastry sheet
- 3 tbsp light brown sugar
- 2 tsp ground cinnamon
- 2 tsp butter, melted
- For the Icing:
- ¼ tsp vanilla extract
- ¼ tsp salt
- 2 tbsp milk
- 1 tbsp lemon zest
- ¼ cup confectioners' sugar

Directions:

1. Preheat your air fryer to 320°F (160°C).
2. In a small bowl, mix together the brown sugar and ground cinnamon. Set this cinnamon sugar mixture aside.
3. Unroll the puff pastry sheet on its paper and brush the entire surface with the melted butter.
4. Sprinkle the cinnamon sugar mixture evenly over the buttered pastry sheet.
5. Roll up the pastry sheet tightly, creating a log. Make sure the seam is sealed.
6. Cut the rolled pastry into 1-inch wide slices to form cinnamon rolls.
7. Place the cinnamon rolls with the spiral side facing up into a greased baking pan.
8. Carefully transfer the baking pan with the cinnamon rolls into the air fryer basket.
9. Air-fry the cinnamon rolls at 320°F for approximately 18-20 minutes, or until they are golden brown and cooked through.
10. Once the cinnamon rolls are done, remove them from the air fryer and allow them to cool for 5-10 minutes.
11. While the cinnamon rolls are cooling, prepare the icing. In a small bowl, combine the softened mascarpone cheese, vanilla extract, and salt. Whisk until the mixture is smooth and creamy.
12. Gradually add confectioners' sugar to the mascarpone mixture, continuing to whisk until fully blended.
13. To achieve the desired consistency for your icing, slowly add milk, one teaspoon at a time, until the glaze is pourable but still has some thickness.
14. Drizzle the icing over the warm cinnamon rolls while they are still in the baking pan.
15. Scatter lemon zest over the top of the cinnamon rolls to add a zesty twist.
16. Serve the Mascarpone Iced Cinnamon Rolls while they are still warm and enjoy!

Eggless Mung Bean Tart

Servings: 2

Cooking Time: 20 Minutes

Ingredients:

- 10 ml soy sauce
- 5 ml lime juice
- 1 large garlic clove, minced or pressed
- 2.5 ml red chili flakes
- 120 grams mung beans, soaked
- Salt and pepper to taste
- 1/2 minced shallot
- 1 green onion, chopped

Directions:

1. Preheat the air fryer to 200°C (390°F).
2. In a bowl, add the soy sauce, lime juice, minced garlic, and red chili flakes. Stir to combine, then set aside.
3. Place the drained mung beans in a blender along with 120 ml (1/2 cup) of water. Season with salt and pepper to taste. Blend until the mixture becomes smooth.
4. Stir in the minced shallot and chopped green onion into the blended mung bean mixture. Do not blend them.
5. Pour the batter into a greased baking pan.
6. Bake the mung bean tart in the air fryer for 15 minutes or until it turns golden. You can check the doneness by inserting a knife into the center; it should come out clean.
7. Once cooked, cut the "quiche" into quarters.
8. Drizzle the prepared sauce over the tart and serve.

Canadian Bacon & Cheese Sandwich

Servings: 1

Cooking Time: 30 Minutes

Ingredients:

- 1 English muffin, halved
- 1 egg
- 1 slice of Canadian bacon
- 1 slice of provolone cheese

Directions:

1. Preheat the air fryer to 180°C (350°F).
2. Place the English muffin halves, crusty side up, in the air fryer basket.
3. Lay a slice of Canadian bacon next to the muffins.
4. Air fry for 5 minutes.
5. Flip the bacon and muffins, and place a slice of provolone cheese on top of the muffins.
6. Beat the egg in a small heatproof bowl.
7. Add the bowl to the air fryer basket next to the bacon and muffins.
8. Air fry for an additional 15 minutes, or until the cheese has melted, the bacon is crispy, and the egg is set.
9. Remove the toasted muffin halves to a plate.
10. Layer a slice of Canadian bacon, then the egg, and top with the second toasted muffin half.

Herby Parmesan Pita

Servings: 2

Cooking Time: 15 Minutes

Ingredients:

- 1 whole-wheat pita
- 10ml (2 tsp) olive oil
- 30g sweet onion, diced
- 1 clove garlic, minced
- 1 egg
- 0.25g dried tarragon
- 0.25g dried thyme
- A pinch of salt
- 9g grated Parmesan cheese

Directions:

1. Preheat the air fryer to 190°C (380°F).
2. Lightly brush the top of the pita with olive oil, then top with diced onion and minced garlic.
3. Crack the egg into a small bowl and sprinkle it with tarragon, thyme, and a pinch of salt.
4. Place the pita in the air fryer frying basket and gently pour the seasoned egg onto the top of the pita.
5. Sprinkle grated Parmesan cheese over the top.
6. Bake for 6 minutes in the preheated air fryer.
7. Allow the pita to cool for 5 minutes, then cut it into pieces and serve.

Cheddar & Egg Scramble

Servings: 4

Cooking Time: 20 Minutes

Ingredients:

- 8 eggs
- 60ml buttermilk
- 60ml milk
- Salt and pepper to taste
- 3 tablespoons butter, melted
- 120g grated cheddar
- 1 tablespoon minced parsley

Directions:

1. Preheat the air fryer to 180°C (350°F).
2. Whisk the eggs with buttermilk, milk, salt, and pepper until foamy and set aside.
3. Put the melted butter in a cake pan and pour in the egg mixture.
4. Return the pan to the fryer and cook for 7 minutes, stirring occasionally.
5. Stir in the cheddar cheese and cook for 2-4 more minutes or until the eggs have set.
6. Remove the cake pan and scoop the eggs onto a serving plate.
7. Scatter with freshly minced parsley and serve.

Effortless Toffee Zucchini Bread

Servings: 6

Cooking Time: 30 Minutes

Ingredients:

- 120 grams flour
- 1/2 tsp baking soda
- 100 grams granulated sugar
- 1/4 tsp ground cinnamon
- 1/4 tsp nutmeg
- 1/4 tsp salt
- 85 grams grated zucchini
- 1 large egg
- 15 ml olive oil
- 5 ml vanilla extract
- 30 grams English toffee bits
- 30 grams mini chocolate chips
- 60 grams chopped walnuts

Directions:

1. Preheat the air fryer to 190°C (375°F).
2. In a bowl, combine the flour, baking soda, toffee bits, granulated sugar, ground cinnamon, nutmeg, salt, grated zucchini, egg, olive oil, vanilla extract, and chocolate chips.
3. Add the chopped walnuts to the batter and mix until they are evenly distributed.
4. Grease a cake pan.
5. Pour the batter into the greased cake pan.
6. Place the cake pan in the air fryer.
7. Bake for 20 minutes or until a toothpick inserted into the center comes out clean.
8. Allow the bread to sit for 10 minutes until it has slightly cooled.
9. Slice and serve immediately.

Ham And Cheddar Gritters

Servings: 6

Cooking Time: 12 Minutes

Ingredients:

- 950 ml water
- 190 g quick-cooking grits
- 1/4 teaspoon salt
- 30 g butter
- 190 g grated Cheddar cheese, divided
- 140 g finely diced ham
- 15 g chopped chives
- Salt and freshly ground black pepper
- 1 egg, beaten
- 160 g panko breadcrumbs
- Vegetable oil

Directions:

1. Bring the water to a boil in a saucepan. Whisk in the grits and 1/4 teaspoon of salt, and cook for 7 minutes until the grits are soft. Remove the pan from the heat and stir in the butter and 140 g of the grated Cheddar cheese. Transfer the grits to a bowl and let them cool for just 10 to 15 minutes.
2. Stir the ham, chives, and the rest of the cheese into the grits and season with salt and pepper to taste. Add the beaten egg and refrigerate the mixture for 30 minutes. (Try not to chill the grits much longer than 30 minutes, or the mixture will be too firm to shape into patties.)
3. While the grit mixture is chilling, make the country gravy and set it aside.
4. Place the panko breadcrumbs in a shallow dish. Measure out 1/4-cup portions of the grits mixture and shape them into patties. Coat all sides of the patties with the panko breadcrumbs, patting them with your hands so the crumbs adhere to the patties. You should have about 16 patties. Spray both sides of the patties with oil.
5. Preheat the air fryer to 200°C (400°F).
6. In batches of 5 or 6, air-fry the fritters for 8 minutes. Using a flat spatula, flip the fritters over and air-fry for another 4 minutes.
7. Serve hot with country gravy.

All-in-one Breakfast Toast

Servings: 1

Cooking Time: 10 Minutes

Ingredients:

- 1 strip of bacon, diced
- 1 slice of 2.5 cm (1-inch) thick bread (e.g., Texas Toast or hand-sliced bread)
- 15 grams (1 tablespoon) softened butter (optional)
- 1 egg
- Salt and freshly ground black pepper
- 30 grams (1/4 cup) grated Colby or Jack cheese

Directions:

1. Preheat your air fryer to 200°C (400°F).
2. Air-fry the diced bacon for 3 minutes, shaking the basket once or twice during cooking. Once done, transfer the bacon to a plate lined with paper towels and set it aside.
3. Use a sharp paring knife to create a large circle in the middle of the slice of bread. Cut halfway through the bread but not all the way to the cutting board. Press down on the center of the bread slice to form an indentation. If desired, spread the softened butter on the edges and within the hole of the bread.
4. Carefully place the slice of bread in the air fryer basket with the hole facing upwards.
5. Crack the egg into the center of the bread, and season it with salt and pepper.
6. Air-fry at 190°C (380°F) for 5 minutes. Sprinkle the grated cheese around the edges of the bread, leaving the center of the yolk uncovered. Top the cheese with the cooked bacon. Gently press the cheese and bacon into the bread to secure them and prevent them from moving around in the air fryer.
7. Air-fry for an additional one or two minutes, depending on your preference for the doneness of the egg. This step will melt the cheese and complete the cooking of the egg.

Crustless Broccoli, Roasted Pepper, And Fontina Quiche

Servings: 4

Cooking Time: 60 Minutes

Ingredients:

- 18 cm (7-inch) cake pan
- 150 grams broccoli florets
- 180 grams chopped roasted red peppers
- 150 grams grated Fontina cheese
- 6 large eggs
- 180 ml heavy cream
- 1/2 teaspoon salt
- Freshly ground black pepper

Directions:

1. Preheat the air fryer to 180°C (360°F).
2. Grease the inside of a 18 cm (7-inch) cake pan that is at least 10 cm (4 inches) deep or use another oven-safe pan that fits into your air fryer.
3. Place the broccoli florets and chopped roasted red peppers in the cake pan and top them with the grated Fontina cheese.
4. In a bowl, whisk together the large eggs and heavy cream. Season the egg mixture with salt and freshly ground black pepper.
5. Pour the seasoned egg mixture over the cheese and vegetables in the cake pan.
6. Cover the pan with aluminum foil.
7. Transfer the cake pan to the air fryer basket.
8. Air-fry at 180°C (360°F) for 60 minutes. Remove the aluminum foil for the last two minutes of cooking time.
9. Carefully unmold the quiche onto a platter and cut it into slices.
10. Serve the Crustless Broccoli, Roasted Pepper, and Fontina Quiche with a side salad or air-fried potatoes if desired.

Huevos Rancheros

Servings: 4

Cooking Time: 45 Minutes + Cooling Time

Ingredients:

- 1 tbsp olive oil
- 20 cherry tomatoes, halved
- 2 plum tomatoes, chopped
- ¼ cup tomato sauce
- 2 scallions, sliced
- 2 garlic cloves, minced
- 1 tsp honey
- ½ tsp salt
- ⅛ tsp cayenne pepper
- ¼ tsp grated nutmeg
- ¼ tsp paprika
- 4 eggs

Directions:

1. Preheat your air fryer to 370°F (188°C).
2. In a 7-inch springform pan that has been wrapped in foil to prevent leaks, combine the olive oil, cherry tomatoes, chopped plum tomatoes, tomato sauce, scallions, minced garlic, honey, salt, paprika, cayenne pepper, and grated nutmeg.
3. Place the pan in the frying basket of the air fryer.
4. Air fry the mixture for 15-20 minutes, stirring it twice during cooking, until the tomatoes are soft and the sauce has thickened. You can also use a fork to mash some of the tomatoes into the sauce.
5. Break the eggs into the tomato sauce, distributing them evenly.
6. Return the pan to the air fryer and air fry for an additional 2 minutes to cook the eggs. Make sure not to mix them in completely; you want the yolks intact.
7. Continue cooking for an additional 4-8 minutes, or until the eggs are set to your desired level of doneness.
8. Once done, remove the pan from the air fryer and allow it to cool slightly before serving.
9. Serve your delicious Huevos Rancheros directly from the pan and enjoy!

Egg And Sausage Crescent Rolls

Servings: 8

Cooking Time: 11 Minutes

Ingredients:

- 5 large eggs
- 1/4 teaspoon black pepper
- 1/4 teaspoon salt
- 15 ml milk
- 60 grams shredded cheddar cheese
- One 8-ounce package refrigerated crescent rolls
- 60 ml pesto sauce
- 8 fully cooked breakfast sausage links, defrosted

Directions:

1. Preheat the air fryer to 160°C (320°F).
2. In a medium bowl, crack the eggs and whisk them with the black pepper, salt, and milk.
3. Pour the egg mixture into a frying pan over medium heat and scramble the eggs. Just before the eggs are fully cooked, turn off the heat and add in the shredded cheddar cheese. Continue to cook until the cheese has melted and the eggs are done, which should take about 5 minutes in total. Remove from the heat.
4. Remove the crescent rolls from the package and press them flat onto a clean surface lightly dusted with flour.
5. Spread 1 1/2 teaspoons of pesto sauce across the center of each crescent roll.
6. Place equal portions of scrambled eggs across all 8 rolls.
7. Top each roll with a breakfast sausage link and roll the dough up tightly so that it resembles the crescent-roll shape.
8. Lightly spray your air fryer basket with olive oil mist and place the rolls on top.
9. Bake for 6 minutes or until the tops of the rolls are lightly browned.
10. Remove the rolls and let them cool for 3 to 5 minutes before serving.

American Biscuits

Servings: 4

Cooking Time: 30 Minutes

Ingredients:

- 240 grams all-purpose flour
- 15 milliliters baking powder
- 2.5 milliliters baking soda
- 2.5 milliliters cornstarch
- 2.5 milliliters salt
- 2.5 milliliters sugar
- 60 grams cold butter, cubed
- 300 milliliters buttermilk
- 2.5 milliliters vanilla extract
- 5 grams finely crushed walnuts

Directions:

1. Preheat your air fryer to 180°C (350°F).
2. In a mixing bowl, combine the all-purpose flour, baking powder, baking soda, cornstarch, salt, and sugar.
3. Add the cold, cubed butter to the dry ingredients and incorporate it until the mixture resembles coarse crumbs.
4. Gradually stir in the buttermilk and vanilla extract, mixing until a sticky dough forms.
5. With floured hands, divide the dough into 8 equal portions and shape them into balls.
6. Grease a pizza pan and arrange the dough balls on it.
7. Place the pizza pan in the air fryer basket.
8. Air fry for approximately 8 minutes or until the biscuits are golden brown and cooked through.
9. Sprinkle the finely crushed walnuts over the biscuits during the last minute of cooking for added flavor and texture.
10. Serve your delicious American biscuits immediately while they're warm.

Healthy Granola

Servings: 4

Cooking Time: 10 Minutes

Ingredients:

- 60g chocolate hazelnut spread
- 100g chopped pecans
- 100g quick-cooking oats
- 15g chia seeds
- 15g flaxseed
- 15g sesame seeds
- 85g coconut shreds
- 60ml maple syrup
- 15g light brown sugar
- 2.5ml (1/2 tsp) vanilla extract
- 30g hazelnut flour
- 10g cocoa powder
- Salt to taste

Directions:

1. Preheat the air fryer to 175°C (350°F).
2. In a bowl, combine the pecans, oats, chia seeds, flaxseed, sesame seeds, coconut shreds, chocolate hazelnut spread, maple syrup, sugar, vanilla extract, hazelnut flour, cocoa powder, and salt.
3. Press the mixture into a greased cake pan.
4. Place the cake pan in the air fryer basket and bake for 5 minutes, stirring once during cooking.
5. Let the granola cool completely before crumbling it.
6. Store the granola in an airtight container for up to 5 days.

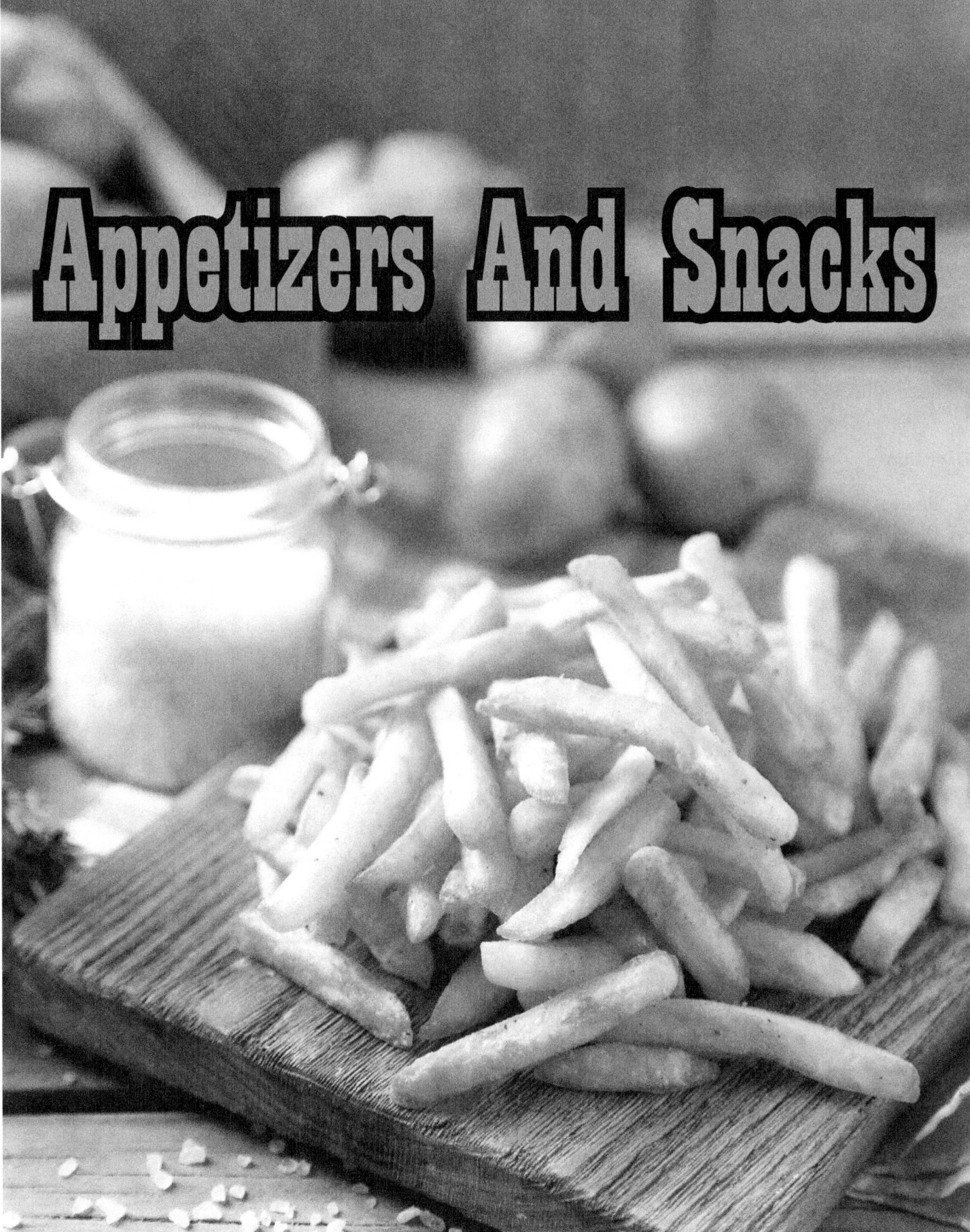

Appetizers And Snacks

Appetizers And Snacks

Corn Dog Bites

Servings: 3

Cooking Time: 12 Minutes

Ingredients:

- 240g Purchased cornbread stuffing mix
- 40g All-purpose flour
- 2 Large eggs, well beaten
- 3 Hot dogs, cut into 5cm pieces (vegetarian hot dogs, if preferred)
- Vegetable oil spray

Directions:

1. Preheat the air fryer to 190°C (375°F).
2. Put the cornbread stuffing mix in a food processor. Cover and pulse to grind into a mixture like fine bread crumbs.
3. Set up and fill three shallow soup plates or small pie plates on your counter: one for the flour, one for the beaten eggs, and one for the stuffing mix crumbs.
4. Dip a hot dog piece in the flour to coat it completely, then gently shake off any excess. Dip the hot dog piece into the beaten eggs and gently roll it around to coat all surfaces. Set the hot dog piece in the stuffing mix crumbs and roll it gently to coat it evenly and well on all sides, including the ends. Set it aside on a cutting board and continue dipping and coating the remaining hot dog pieces.
5. Give the coated hot dog pieces a generous coating of vegetable oil spray on all sides, then set them in the basket in one layer with some space between them.
6. Air-fry undisturbed for 10 minutes, or until golden brown and crunchy. (You may need to add 2 minutes in the air fryer if the temperature is at 180°C.)
7. Use a nonstick-safe spatula, and perhaps a flatware fork for balance, to transfer the corn dog bites to a wire rack. Cool for 5 minutes before serving.

Indian Cauliflower Tikka Bites

Servings: 6

Cooking Time: 20 Minutes

Ingredients:

- 240ml plain Greek yogurt
- 5ml (1 teaspoon) fresh ginger
- 5ml (1 teaspoon) minced garlic
- 5ml (1 teaspoon) vindaloo
- 2.5ml (½ teaspoon) cardamom
- 2.5ml (½ teaspoon) paprika
- 2.5ml (½ teaspoon) turmeric powder
- 2.5ml (½ teaspoon) cumin powder
- 1 large head of cauliflower, washed and cut into medium-size florets
- 120ml panko breadcrumbs
- 1 lemon, quartered
- Instructions:
- Preheat your air fryer to 175°C (350°F).
- In a large bowl, mix together the Greek yogurt, fresh ginger, minced garlic, vindaloo, cardamom, paprika, turmeric powder, and cumin powder.
- Add the cauliflower florets to the bowl, and thoroughly coat them with the yogurt mixture.
- Remove the cauliflower florets from the bowl and place them on a baking sheet. Sprinkle the panko breadcrumbs evenly over the top.
- Place the coated cauliflower bites into the air fryer basket, ensuring there's space between the florets. Depending on the size of your air fryer, you may need to cook in multiple batches.
- Cook the cauliflower for 10 minutes, shake the basket, and continue cooking for an additional 10 minutes or until the florets are lightly browned.
- Remove the cooked cauliflower from the air fryer and keep them warm. Repeat the cooking process until all the cauliflower florets are done.
- Just before serving, lightly squeeze lemon juice over the top of the cauliflower bites.
- Serve the Indian Cauliflower Tikka Bites while they are still warm.

Cholula Avocado Fries

Servings: 2

Cooking Time: 20 Minutes

Ingredients:

- 1 egg, beaten
- 30g flour
- 10g ground flaxseed
- 1.25ml Cholula sauce
- Salt to taste
- 1 avocado, cut into fries

Directions:

1. Preheat the air fryer to 190°C (375°F).
2. Mix the beaten egg and Cholula sauce in a bowl.
3. In another bowl, combine the remaining ingredients, except for the avocado.
4. Submerge the avocado slices in the egg mixture and dredge them into the flour mixture to coat evenly.
5. Place the avocado fries in the lightly greased air fryer basket.
6. Air fry for 5 minutes or until they are golden and crispy.
7. Serve your Cholula Avocado Fries immediately.

Chicken Shawarma Bites

Servings: 6

Cooking Time: 22 Minutes

Ingredients:

- 680g Boneless skinless chicken thighs, trimmed of any fat and cut into 2.5cm pieces
- 22.5ml Olive oil
- Up to 22.5ml Minced garlic
- 2.5g Table salt
- 1.25g Ground cardamom
- 1.25g Ground cinnamon
- 1.25g Ground cumin
- 1.25g Mild paprika
- Up to 1.25g Grated nutmeg
- 1.25g Ground black pepper

Directions:

1. Preheat the air fryer to 200°C (400°F).
2. Mix all the ingredients in a large bowl until the chicken is thoroughly and evenly coated in the oil and spices.
3. When the air fryer reaches the desired temperature, scrape the coated chicken pieces into the basket and spread them out into one layer as much as possible.
4. Air-fry for 22 minutes, shaking the basket at least three times during cooking to rearrange the pieces, until the chicken is well browned and crisp.
5. Pour the chicken pieces onto a wire rack and cool for 5 minutes before serving.

Asian Five-spice Wings

Servings: 4

Cooking Time: 15 Minutes

Ingredients:

- 907 grams chicken wings
- 120 ml Asian-style salad dressing
- 30 ml Chinese five-spice powder

Directions:

1. Begin by cutting off the wing tips and discard them or save them for making stock. Then, cut the remaining wing pieces in two at the joint.
2. Place the wing pieces in a large sealable plastic bag. Pour in the Asian dressing, seal the bag, and massage the marinade into the wings until they are well coated. Refrigerate for at least an hour to marinate.
3. After marinating, remove the wings from the bag, drain off any excess marinade, and place the wings in the air fryer basket.
4. Cook the wings at 180°C (360°F) for 15 minutes or until the juices run clear. About halfway through the cooking time, shake the basket or stir the wings for more even cooking.
5. Transfer the cooked wings to a plate in a single layer.
6. Sprinkle half of the Chinese five-spice powder on one side of the wings, then turn them over and sprinkle the other side with the remaining seasoning.

Chinese-style Potstickers

Servings: 6

Cooking Time: 30 Minutes

Ingredients:

- 240g shredded Chinese cabbage
- 60g chopped shiitake mushrooms
- 60g grated carrots
- 30ml minced chives
- 2 garlic cloves, minced
- 10g grated fresh ginger
- 12 dumpling wrappers
- 10ml sesame oil

Directions:

1. Preheat the air fryer to 190°C (370°F).
2. Toss the Chinese cabbage, shiitake mushrooms, carrots, chives, garlic, and ginger in a baking pan and stir.
3. Place the pan in the air fryer and bake for 3-6 minutes until the vegetables are slightly softened.
4. Put a dumpling wrapper on a clean workspace, then top with a tablespoon of the vegetable mix.
5. Fold the wrapper in half to form a half-circle and use water to seal the edges. Repeat with the remaining wrappers and filling.
6. Brush the potstickers with sesame oil and arrange them on the air fryer basket.
7. Air fry for 5 minutes until the bottoms are golden brown.
8. Take the pan out, add 15ml (1 tablespoon) of water, and put it back in the air fryer to air fry for 4-6 minutes longer until the potstickers are cooked through.
9. Serve your Chinese-Style Potstickers hot.

Beet Chips

Servings: 4

Cooking Time: 20 Minutes

Ingredients:

- 2 large red beets, washed and skinned
- 15 ml avocado oil
- 1/4 teaspoon salt

Directions:

1. Preheat the air fryer to 165°C.
2. Using a mandolin or a sharp knife, slice the beets into 3 mm (1/8-inch) thick slices. Place the beet slices in a bowl of water and let them soak for 30 minutes. Drain the water and pat the beet slices dry with a paper towel or kitchen cloth.
3. In a medium bowl, toss the beet slices with avocado oil and sprinkle them with salt.
4. Lightly spray the air fryer basket with olive oil mist and place the beet chips into the basket. To allow for even cooking, do not overlap the beet slices; cook in batches if necessary.
5. Cook the beet chips for 15 to 20 minutes, shaking the basket every 5 minutes, until the outer edges of the beets begin to flip up like a chip.
6. Remove the beet chips from the basket and serve them warm. Repeat with the remaining beet slices until they are all cooked.

Cocktail Beef Bites

Servings: 4

Cooking Time: 30 Minutes

Ingredients:

- 450g sirloin tip, cubed
- 240ml cheese pasta sauce
- 180g soft bread crumbs
- 30ml olive oil
- 2.5ml garlic powder
- 2.5ml dried thyme

Directions:

1. Preheat the air fryer to 180°C (360°F).
2. Toss the beef and the pasta sauce in a medium bowl. Set aside.
3. In a shallow bowl, mix bread crumbs, oil, garlic, and thyme until well combined.
4. Drop the cubes in the crumb mixture to coat.
5. Place them in the greased frying basket and bake for 6-8 minutes, shaking once until the beef is crisp and browned.
6. Serve warm with cocktail forks or toothpicks.

Classic Potato Chips

Servings: 4

Cooking Time: 8 Minutes

Ingredients:

- 2 medium russet potatoes, washed
- 473 ml filtered water
- 15 ml avocado oil
- 2.5 ml salt

Directions:

1. Using a mandolin, slice the potatoes into 3 mm-thick pieces.
2. Pour the water into a large bowl. Place the potatoes in the bowl and soak for at least 30 minutes.
3. Preheat the air fryer to 175°C (350°F).
4. Drain the water and pat the potatoes dry with a paper towel or kitchen cloth. Toss with avocado oil and salt.
5. Liberally spray the air fryer basket with olive oil mist.
6. Set the potatoes inside the air fryer basket, separating them so they're not on top of each other.
7. Cook for 5 minutes, shake the basket, and cook for another 5 minutes, or until browned.
8. Remove and let cool a few minutes prior to serving. Repeat until all the chips are cooked.

Buffalo Bites

Servings: 16

Cooking Time: 12 Minutes

Ingredients:

- 450 grams ground chicken
- 4 tablespoons buffalo wing sauce
- 56 grams Gruyère cheese, cut into 16 cubes
- 15 ml maple syrup

Directions:

1. Mix 2 tablespoons of buffalo wing sauce into the ground chicken.
2. Shape the chicken mixture into a log and divide it into 16 equal portions.
3. With slightly damp hands, mold each portion of chicken around a cube of Gruyère cheese and shape it into a firm ball.
4. When you have shaped 8 meatballs, place them in the air fryer basket.
5. Cook at 200°C (390°F) for approximately 5 minutes. Shake the basket, reduce the temperature to 180°C (360°F), and cook for an additional 5 minutes.
6. While the first batch is cooking, shape the remaining chicken and cheese into 8 more meatballs.
7. Repeat step 5 to cook the second batch of meatballs.
8. In a medium bowl, mix the remaining 2 tablespoons of buffalo wing sauce with the maple syrup. Add all the cooked meatballs and toss to coat.
9. Place the meatballs back into the air fryer basket and cook at 200°C (390°F) for 2 minutes to set the glaze.
10. Skewer each meatball with a toothpick and serve.

Black-olive Poppers

Servings: 5

Cooking Time: 20 Minutes

Ingredients:

- 5 jalapeño peppers, cut lengthwise, seeded
- 60 ml cream cheese, softened
- 60 ml grated cheddar
- 15 ml chopped black olives
- 15 ml chopped green olives
- 5 ml dried oregano
- 15 ml mayonnaise
- 15 ml Parmesan cheese
- 15 ml dried parsley

Directions:

1. Preheat the air fryer to 180°C (350°F).
2. Mix all ingredients, except for the jalapeño peppers, in a bowl.
3. Add the prepared mixture into each jalapeño half.
4. Lay the stuffed peppers in the air fryer basket.
5. Bake for 8 minutes in the preheated air fryer.
6. Transfer the jalapeño poppers to a serving plate.
7. Serve them right away and sprinkle with dried parsley.

Cauliflower "tater" Tots

Servings: 6

Cooking Time: 10 Minutes

Ingredients:

- 1 head of cauliflower
- 2 eggs
- 30g all-purpose flour*
- 125g grated Parmesan cheese
- 1 teaspoon salt
- Freshly ground black pepper
- Vegetable or olive oil, in a spray bottle

Directions:

1. Grate the head of cauliflower with a box grater or finely chop it in a food processor. You should have about 875ml (3½ cups) of grated cauliflower.
2. Place the chopped cauliflower in the center of a clean kitchen towel and twist the towel tightly to squeeze all the water out of the cauliflower. You may need to do this in two batches to ensure all the water is removed.
3. Transfer the squeezed cauliflower to a large bowl. Add the eggs, all-purpose flour, grated Parmesan cheese, salt, and freshly ground black pepper. Mix well until all the ingredients are combined.
4. Shape the cauliflower mixture into small cylinders or "tater tot" shapes, rolling roughly one tablespoon of the mixture at a time. Place the tots on a cookie sheet lined with paper towels to absorb any residual moisture.
5. Spray the cauliflower tots all over with vegetable or olive oil using an oil spray bottle.
6. Preheat the air fryer to 200°C (400°F).
7. Air-fry the tots at 200°C (400°F), in a single layer, for 10 minutes, turning them over for the last few minutes of the cooking process to ensure even browning.
8. Season the cauliflower tots with salt and black pepper to taste.
9. Serve the "Tater" Tots hot with your favorite dipping sauce.

Buffalo Wings

Servings: 2

Cooking Time: 12 Minutes Per Batch

Ingredients:

- 900 grams chicken wings
- 45 ml butter, melted
- 60 ml hot sauce (like Crystal® or Frank's®)
- Finishing Sauce:
- 45 ml butter, melted
- 60 ml hot sauce (like Crystal® or Frank's®)
- 5 ml Worcestershire sauce

Directions:

1. Prepare the chicken wings by cutting off the wing tips and discarding (or freezing for chicken stock). Divide the drumettes from the wingettes by cutting through the joint. Place the chicken wing pieces in a large bowl.
2. Combine the melted butter and the hot sauce and stir to blend well. Pour the marinade over the chicken wings, cover, and let the wings marinate for 2 hours or up to overnight in the refrigerator.
3. Preheat the air fryer to 200°C (400°F).
4. Air-fry the wings in two batches for 10 minutes per batch, shaking the basket halfway through the cooking process. When both batches are done, toss all the wings back into the basket for another 2 minutes to heat through and finish cooking.
5. While the wings are air-frying, combine the remaining 45 ml of butter, 60 ml of hot sauce, and the Worcestershire sauce.
6. Remove the wings from the air fryer, toss them in the finishing sauce, and serve with some cooling blue cheese dip and celery sticks.

Charred Shishito Peppers

Servings: 4

Cooking Time: 5 Minutes

Ingredients:

- 20 shishito peppers (about 170g)
- 5ml vegetable oil
- Coarse sea salt
- 1 lemon

Directions:

1. Preheat the air fryer to 200°C (390°F).
2. Toss the shishito peppers with the vegetable oil and a sprinkle of coarse sea salt. You can do this in a bowl or directly in the air fryer basket.
3. Air-fry the shishito peppers at 200°C (390°F) for 5 minutes, shaking the basket once or twice during the cooking process to ensure even cooking.
4. Turn the charred peppers out into a bowl.
5. Squeeze some lemon juice over the top and season with coarse sea salt.
6. These should be served as finger foods - pick the pepper up by the stem and eat the whole pepper, seeds and all. Be cautious, as occasionally, you might encounter a spicy one!

Cheddar Stuffed Pepper

Servings: 5

Cooking Time: 15 Minutes

Ingredients:

- 10 jalapeño peppers
- 170g ricotta cheese
- 60g grated cheddar cheese
- 30ml bread crumbs

Directions:

1. Preheat the air fryer to 170°C (340°F).
2. Cut the jalapeño peppers in half lengthwise and carefully remove the seeds and membrane. Set them aside.
3. Microwave the ricotta cheese in a small bowl for 15 seconds to soften it. Stir in the grated cheddar cheese to combine.
4. Stuff each jalapeño half with the cheese mixture.
5. Top the stuffed jalapeños with bread crumbs.
6. Place the stuffed jalapeños in the air fryer basket and lightly spray them with cooking oil.
7. Air fry the jalapeños for 5-6 minutes, or until they are heated through and the bread crumbs are golden.
8. Serve the Cheddar Stuffed Jalapeños warm.

Artichoke Samosas

Servings: 6

Cooking Time: 25 Minutes

Ingredients:

- 125 grams minced artichoke hearts
- 60 grams ricotta cheese
- 1 egg white
- 3 tablespoons grated mozzarella
- ½ teaspoon dried thyme
- 6 sheets of filo pastry
- 2 tablespoons melted butter
- 240 ml mango chutney

Directions:

1. Preheat the air fryer to 200°C (400°F).
2. In a small bowl, mix together the ricotta cheese, egg white, minced artichoke hearts, grated mozzarella cheese, and dried thyme until well blended.
3. When you take out the filo pastry sheets, cover them with a damp kitchen towel to prevent them from drying out while you work with them.
4. Take one sheet of filo pastry and place it on the work surface. Cut it into thirds lengthwise.
5. At the base of each strip, place about 1 ½ teaspoons of the filling.
6. Fold the bottom right-hand corner of the strip over to the left-hand side to create a triangle. Continue folding and forming triangles along the strip.
7. Brush the triangle with melted butter to seal the edges.
8. Place the prepared triangles in the greased frying basket of the air fryer.
9. Bake until the samosas are golden and crisp, which should take approximately 4 minutes.
10. Serve the Artichoke Samosas with mango chutney.

Air Fryer Cookbook

Baba Ghanouj

Servings: 2

Cooking Time: 40 Minutes

Ingredients:

- 2 small (340 grams each) purple Italian eggplants
- 60 ml Olive oil
- 60 ml Tahini
- 1/2 teaspoon Ground black pepper
- 1/4 teaspoon Onion powder
- 1/4 teaspoon Mild smoked paprika (optional)
- Up to 1 teaspoon Table salt

Directions:

1. Preheat the air fryer to 200°C (400°F).
2. Prick the eggplants on all sides with a fork. Once the air fryer has reached the desired temperature, place the eggplants in the basket in one layer. Air-fry them undisturbed for 40 minutes, or until they become blackened and soft.
3. Remove the basket from the air fryer. Allow the eggplants to cool in the basket for 20 minutes.
4. Use a nonstick-safe spatula, and perhaps a flatware tablespoon for balance, to gently transfer the eggplants to a bowl. The juices will run out, so make sure the bowl is close to the basket. Split the eggplants open.
5. Scrape the soft insides of half an eggplant into a food processor. Repeat this process with the remaining piece(s). Add any juices from the bowl to the eggplant in the food processor, but discard the skins and stems.
6. Add the olive oil, tahini, ground black pepper, onion powder, and smoked paprika (if using). Start by adding about half of the salt. Then, cover and process until smooth, stopping the machine at least once to scrape down the inside of the canister. Taste the spread for salt and add more as needed.
7. Scrape the baba ghanouj into a bowl and serve it warm, or set it aside at room temperature for up to 2 hours. You can also cover and store it in the refrigerator for up to 4 days.

Hot Garlic Kale Chips

Servings: 6

Cooking Time: 20 Minutes

Ingredients:

- 1 tbsp chili powder
- 1 tsp garlic powder
- 6 cups kale, torn
- 3 tsp olive oil
- Sea salt to taste

Directions:

1. Preheat your air fryer to 199°C (390°F).
2. In a small bowl, mix together the chili powder and garlic powder.
3. Tear the kale into bite-sized pieces and place them in a large mixing bowl.
4. Drizzle the torn kale with olive oil and toss to evenly coat the kale leaves.
5. Sprinkle the chili and garlic powder mixture over the kale and toss again to make sure the seasoning is distributed evenly.
6. Grease the air fryer basket to prevent sticking and place the seasoned kale leaves in the basket. It's okay to fill it, but don't overcrowd.
7. Air fry the kale at 199°C (390°F) for about 5-6 minutes. You may want to shake the basket or toss the kale halfway through cooking to ensure even crisping.
8. Keep a close eye on the kale as it can go from crispy to burnt quickly. It should be crispy but not browned.
9. Once the kale chips are done, remove them from the air fryer and immediately sprinkle with sea salt to taste.
10. Allow the kale chips to cool slightly, and then serve them as a crunchy and flavorful snack.

Cayenne-spiced Roasted Pecans

Servings: 4

Cooking Time: 15 Minutes

Ingredients:

- 1/4 tsp chili powder
- Salt and pepper to taste
- 1/8 tsp cayenne pepper
- 1 tsp cumin powder
- 1 tsp cinnamon powder
- 1/8 tsp garlic powder
- 1/8 tsp onion powder
- 120g raw pecans
- 30g butter, melted
- 5g honey

Directions:

1. Preheat the air fryer to 150°C (300°F).
2. In a bowl, whisk together black pepper, chili powder, salt, cayenne pepper, cumin, garlic powder, cinnamon, and onion powder. Set the spice mixture aside.
3. Toss the raw pecans, melted butter, and honey in a medium bowl until the pecans are well coated.
4. Add the spice mixture to the pecans and toss them to ensure even distribution of the spices.
5. Pour the spiced pecans into the air fryer frying basket.
6. Toast the pecans for 3 minutes, stirring them once during this time.
7. After 3 minutes, stir the pecans again and toast for another 3 to 5 minutes until the nuts are crisp and have a roasted aroma.
8. Allow the roasted pecans to cool before serving.

Individual Pizzas

Servings: 2

Cooking Time: 7 Minutes

Ingredients:

- 170 grams purchased fresh pizza dough (not a prebaked crust)
- Olive oil spray
- 4.5 tablespoons purchased pizza sauce or purchased pesto
- 60 grams (about 2 ounces) shredded semi-firm mozzarella
- Instructions:
- Preheat your air fryer to 200°C (400°F).
- Press the pizza dough into a 13-centimeter (5-inch) circle for a small air fryer, a 15-centimeter (6-inch) circle for a medium air fryer, or an 18-centimeter (7-inch) circle for a large machine. Generously coat the top of the dough with olive oil spray.
- Remove the basket from the air fryer machine and place the dough, oil side down, in the basket. Smear the sauce or pesto evenly over the dough, then sprinkle it with the shredded cheese.
- Return the basket to the air fryer machine and air-fry undisturbed for 7 minutes, or until the dough is puffed, browned, and the cheese has melted. (Adding extra toppings should not increase the cooking time, provided you don't add extra cheese.)
- Remove the basket from the machine and let the pizza cool in it for 5 minutes. Use a large non-stick-safe spatula to transfer the pizza from the basket to a wire rack. Allow it to cool for an additional 5 minutes before serving.

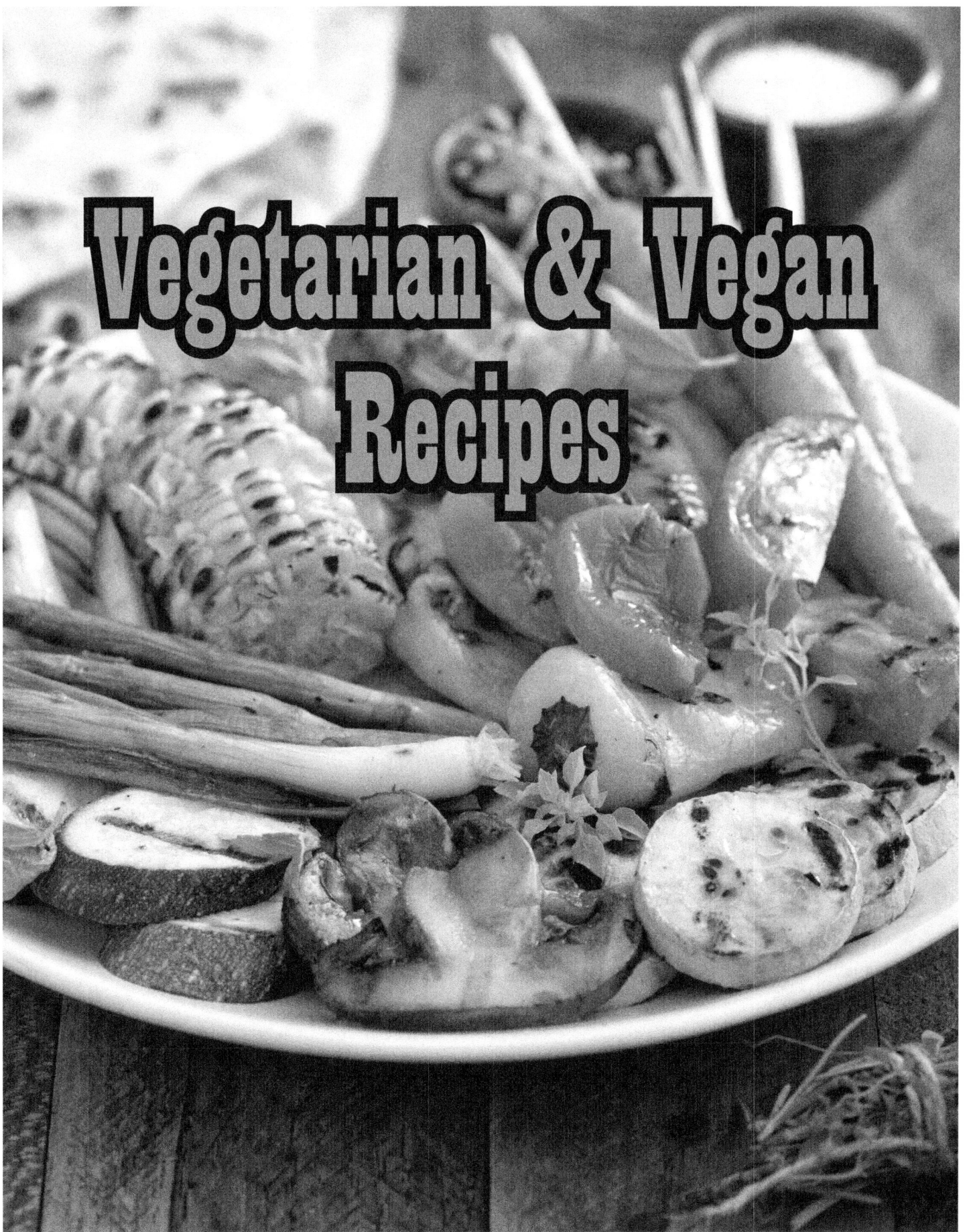

Vegetarian & Vegan Recipes

Roast Cauliflower & Broccoli

Servings: 6

Cooking Time: xx

Ingredients:

- 300g broccoli
- 300g cauliflower
- 2 tbsp oil
- ½ tsp garlic powder
- ¼ tsp salt
- ¼ tsp paprika
- ⅛ tsp pepper

Directions:

1. Preheat air fryer to 200°C
2. Place broccoli and cauliflower in a bowl and microwave for 3 minutes
3. Add remaining ingredients and mix well
4. Add to the air fryer and cook for about 12 mins

Potato Gratin

Servings: 4

Cooking Time: xx

Ingredients:

- 2 large potatoes
- 2 beaten eggs
- 100ml coconut cream
- 1 tbsp plain flour
- 50g grated cheddar

Directions:

1. Slice the potatoes into thin slices, place in the air fryer and cook for 10 minutes at 180°C
2. Mix eggs, coconut cream and flour together
3. Line four ramekins with the potato slices
4. Cover with the cream mixture, sprinkle with cheese and cook for 10 minutes at 200°C

Sweet Potato Taquitos

Servings: 10

Cooking Time: xx

Ingredients:

- 1 sweet potato cut into ½ inch pieces
- 1 ½ tsp oil
- 1 chopped onion
- 1 tsp minced garlic
- 400g black beans
- 3 tbsp water
- 10 corn tortillas
- 1 chipotle pepper, chopped
- ½ tsp cumin
- ½ tsp paprika
- ½ chilli powder
- ⅛ tsp salt
- ½ tsp maple syrup

Directions:

1. Place the sweet potato in the air fryer spray with oil and cook for 12 minutes at 200°C
2. Heat oil in a pan, add the onion and garlic and cook for a few minutes until soft
3. Add remaining ingredients to the pan, add 2 tbsp of water and combine
4. Add the sweet potato and 1 tbsp of water and mix
5. Warm the tortilla in the microwave for about 1 minute
6. Place a row of filling across the centre of each tortilla. Fold up the bottom of the tortilla, tuck under the filling, fold in the edges then continue to roll the tortilla
7. Place in the air fryer and cook for about 12 minutes

Cheese, Tomato & Pesto Crustless Quiches

Servings: 1–2

Cooking Time:xx

Ingredients:

- 40 g/½ cup grated mature Cheddar
- 3 eggs, beaten
- 3 cherry tomatoes, finely chopped
- salt and freshly ground black pepper
- ½ teaspoon olive oil, to grease ramekins
- 2 tablespoons pesto (jarred or see page 80)

Directions:

1. Preheat the air-fryer to 180ºC/350ºF.
2. Mix together the cheese, eggs, tomatoes, salt and pepper in a bowl.
3. Grease the ramekins with the oil (and line with parchment paper if you wish to remove the quiches to serve). Pour the egg mixture into the ramekins.
4. Place the ramekins in the preheated air-fryer and air-fry for 10 minutes, stirring the contents of the ramekins halfway through cooking. Serve hot with 1 tablespoon pesto drizzled over each quiche.

Butternut Squash Fries

Servings: 2

Cooking Time:xx

Ingredients:

- 300g butternut squash, cut into sticks
- 1 tbsp olive oil
- 2 tsp bagel seasoning
- 1 tsp chopped rosemary

Directions:

1. Preheat air fryer to 200ºC
2. Drizzle oil over butternut squash and coat well
3. Add to air fryer and cook for about 20 minutes
4. Sprinkle with seasoning

Bbq Soy Curls

Servings: 2

Cooking Time:xx

Ingredients:

- 250ml warm water
- 1 tsp vegetable bouillon
- 200g soy curls
- 40g BBQ sauce
- 1 tsp oil

Directions:

1. Soak the soy curls in water and bouillon for 10 minutes
2. Place the soy curls in another bowl and shred
3. Heat the air fryer to 200ºC
4. Cook for 3 minutes
5. Remove from the air fryer and coat in bbq sauce
6. Return to the air fryer and cook for 5 minutes shaking halfway through

Spicy Spanish Potatoes

Servings: 2

Cooking Time:xx

Ingredients:

- 4 large potatoes
- 1 tbsp olive oil
- 2 tsp paprika
- 2 tsp dried garlic
- 1 tsp barbacoa seasoning
- Salt and pepper

Directions:

1. Chop the potatoes into wedges
2. Place them in a bowl with olive oil and seasoning, mix well
3. Add to the air fryer and cook at 160ºC for 20 minutes
4. Shake, increase heat to 200ºC and cook for another 3 minutes

Air Fryer Cookbook

Orange Zingy Cauliflower

Servings: 2

Cooking Time: xx

Ingredients:

- 200ml water
- 200g flour
- Half the head of a cauliflower, cut into 1.5" florets
- 2 tsp olive oil
- 2 minced garlic cloves
- 1 tsp minced ginger
- 150ml orange juice
- 3 tbsp white vinegar
- 1/2 tsp red pepper flakes
- 1 tsp sesame oil 100g brown sugar
- 3 tbsp soy sauce
- 1 tbsp cornstarch
- 2 tbsp water
- 1 tsp salt

Directions:

1. Take a medium mixing bowl and add the water, salt and flour together
2. Dip each floret of cauliflower into the mixture and place in the air fryer basket
3. Cook at 220°C for 15 minutes
4. Meanwhile make the orange sauce by combining all ingredients in a saucepan and allowing to simmer for 3 minutes, until the sauce has thickened
5. Drizzle the sauce over the cauliflower to serve

Mini Quiche

Servings: 2

Cooking Time: xx

Ingredients:

- 100g raw cashews
- 3 tbsp milk
- ½ tsp hot sauce
- 1 tsp white miso paste
- 1 tsp mustard
- 300g tofu
- 100g bacon pieces
- 1 chopped red pepper
- 1 chopped onion
- 6 tbsp yeast
- ½ tsp onion powder
- ½ tsp paprika
- ½ tsp cumin
- ½ tsp chilli powder
- ½ tsp black pepper
- ⅛ tsp turmeric
- ½ tsp canola oil
- 50g curly kale

Directions:

1. Heat the oil in a pan, add the bacon pepper, onion and curly kale and cook for about 3 minutes
2. Place all the other ingredients into a blender and blend until smooth
3. Add to a bowl with the bacon, pepper, onion and curly kale and mix well
4. Fill silicone muffin cups with the mix
5. Place in the air fryer and cook at 165°C for 15 minutes

Bagel Pizza

Servings: 1

Cooking Time: xx

Ingredients:

- 1 bagel
- 2 tbsp marinara sauce
- 6 slices vegan pepperoni
- 2 tbsp mozzarella
- Pinch of basil

Directions:

1. Heat the air fryer to 180°C
2. Cut the bagel in half and toast for 2 minutes in the air fryer
3. Remove from the air fryer and top with marinara sauce, pepperoni and mozzarella
4. Return to the air fryer and cook for 4-5 minutes
5. Sprinkle with basil to serve

Ratatouille

Servings: 4

Cooking Time:xx

Ingredients:

- ½ small aubergine, cubed
- 1 courgette, cubed
- 1 tomato, cubed
- 1 pepper, cut into cubes
- ½ onion, diced
- 1 fresh cayenne pepper, sliced
- 1 tsp vinegar
- 5 sprigs basil, chopped
- 2 sprigs oregano, chopped
- 1 clove garlic, crushed
- Salt and pepper
- 1 tbsp olive oil
- 1 tbsp white wine

Directions:

1. Preheat air fryer to 200°C
2. Place all ingredients in a bowl and mix
3. Pour into a baking dish
4. Add dish to the air fryer and cook for 8 minutes, stir then cook for another 10 minutes

Courgette Meatballs

Servings: 4

Cooking Time:xx

Ingredients:

- 400g oats
- 40g feta, crumbled
- 1 beaten egg
- Salt and pepper
- 150g courgette
- 1 tsp lemon rind
- 6 basil leaves, thinly sliced
- 1 tsp dill
- 1 tsp oregano

Directions:

1. Preheat the air fryer to 200°C
2. Grate the courgette into a bowl, squeeze any access water out
3. Add all the remaining ingredients apart from the oats and mix well
4. Blend the oats until they resemble breadcrumbs
5. Add the oats into the other mix and stir well
6. Form into balls and place in the air fryer cook for 10 minutes

Paneer Tikka

Servings: 2

Cooking Time:xx

Ingredients:

- 200ml yogurt
- 1 tsp ginger garlic paste
- 1 tsp red chilli powder
- 1 tsp garam masala
- 1 tsp turmeric powder
- 1 tbsp dried fenugreek leaves
- The juice of 1 lemon
- 2 tbsp chopped coriander
- 1 tbsp olive oil
- 250g paneer cheese, cut into cubes
- 1 green pepper, chopped
- 1 red pepper, chopped
- 1 yellow pepper, chopped
- 1 chopped onion

Directions:

1. Take a mixing bowl and add the yogurt, garlic paste, red chilli powder, garam masala, turmeric powder, lemon juice, fenugreek and chopped coriander, combining well
2. Place the marinade to one side
3. Add the cubed cheese to the marinade and toss to coat well
4. Leave to marinade for 2 hours
5. Take 8 skewers and alternate the cheese with the peppers and onions
6. Drizzle a little oil over the top
7. Arrange in the air fryer and cook at 220°C for 3 minutes
8. Turn and cook for another 3 minutes

Vegan Fried Ravioli

Servings: 4

Cooking Time: xx

Ingredients:

- 100g panko breadcrumbs
- 2 tsp yeast
- 1 tsp basil
- 1 tsp oregano
- 1 tsp garlic powder
- Pinch salt and pepper
- 50ml liquid from can of chickpeas
- 150g vegan ravioli
- Cooking spray
- 50g marinara for dipping

Directions:

1. Combine the breadcrumbs, yeast, basil, oregano, garlic powder and salt and pepper
2. Put the liquid from the chickpeas in a bowl
3. Dip the ravioli in the liquid then dip into the breadcrumb mix
4. Heat the air fryer to 190°C
5. Place the ravioli in the air fryer and cook for about 6 minutes until crispy

Camembert & Soldiers

Servings: 2

Cooking Time: xx

Ingredients:

- 1 piece of Camembert
- 2 slices sandwich bread
- 1 tbsp mustard

Directions:

1. Preheat the air fryer to 180°C
2. Place the camembert in a sturdy container, cook in the air fryer for 15 minutes
3. Toast the bread and cut into soldiers
4. Serve with the mustard by the side

Aubergine Parmigiana

Servings: 2 As A Main Or 4 As A Side

Cooking Time: xx

Ingredients:

- 2 small or 1 large aubergine/eggplant, sliced 5 mm/¼ in. thick
- 1 tablespoon olive oil
- ¾ teaspoon salt
- 200 g/7 oz. mozzarella, sliced
- ½ teaspoon freshly ground black pepper
- 20 g/¼ cup finely grated Parmesan
- green vegetables, to serve
- SAUCE
- 135 g/5 oz. passata/strained tomatoes
- 1 teaspoon dried oregano
- ¼ teaspoon garlic salt
- 1 tablespoon olive oil

Directions:

1. Preheat the air-fryer to 200°C/400°F.
2. Rub each of the aubergine/eggplant slices with olive oil and salt. Divide the slices into two batches. Place one batch of the aubergine slices in the preheated air-fryer and air-fry for 4 minutes on one side, then turn over and air-fry for 2 minutes on the other side. Lay these on the base of a gratin dish that fits into your air-fryer.
3. Air-fry the second batch of aubergine slices in the same way. Whilst they're cooking, mix together the sauce ingredients in a small bowl.
4. Spread the sauce over the aubergines in the gratin dish. Add a layer of the mozzarella slices, then season with pepper. Add a second layer of aubergine slices, then top with Parmesan.
5. Place the gratin dish in the air-fryer and air-fry for 6 minutes, until the mozzarella is melted and the top of the dish is golden brown. Serve immediately with green vegetables on the side.

Spinach And Egg Air Fryer Breakfast Muffins

Servings: 4

Cooking Time: 10 Minutes

Ingredients:

- 8 eggs
- 100 g / 3.5 oz fresh spinach
- 50 g / 1.8 oz cheddar cheese, grated
- ½ onion, finely sliced
- 1 tsp black pepper

Directions:

1. Preheat your air fryer to 200 °C / 400 °F and line an 8-pan muffin tray with parchment paper or grease with olive oil.
2. Gently press the spinach leaves into the bottom of each prepared muffin cup.
3. Sprinkle the finely sliced onion on top of the spinach.
4. Crack 2 eggs into each cup on top of the spinach and add some of the grated cheddar cheese on top of the eggs. Top with a light sprinkle of black pepper.
5. Carefully place the muffins into the air fryer basket and shut the lid. Bake for 10 minutes until the eggs are set and the muffins are hot throughout.
6. Serve the muffins while still hot for breakfast.

Veggie Bakes

Servings: 2

Cooking Time: xx

Ingredients:

- Any type of leftover vegetable bake you have
- 30g flour

Directions:

1. Preheat the air fryer to 180ºC
2. Mix the flour with the leftover vegetable bake
3. Shape into balls and place in the air fryer
4. Cook for 10 minutes

Parmesan Truffle Oil Fries

Servings: 2

Cooking Time: xx

Ingredients:

- 3 large potatoes, peeled and cut
- 2 tbsp truffle oil
- 2 tbsp grated parmesan
- 1 tsp paprika
- 1 tbsp parsley
- Salt and pepper to taste

Directions:

1. Coat the potatoes with truffle oil and sprinkle with seasonings
2. Add the fries to the air fryer
3. Cook at 180ºC for about 15 minutes shake halfway through
4. Sprinkle with parmesan and parsley to serve

Broccoli Cheese

Servings: 2

Cooking Time: xx

Ingredients:

- 250g broccoli
- Cooking spray
- 10 tbsp evaporated milk
- 300g Mexican cheese
- 4 tsp Amarillo paste
- 6 saltine crackers

Directions:

1. Heat the air fryer to 190ºC
2. Place the broccoli in the air fryer spray with cooking oil and cook for about 6 minutes
3. Place the remaining ingredients in a blender and process until smooth
4. Place in a bowl and microwave for 30 seconds
5. Pour over the broccoli and serve

Artichoke Pasta

Servings: 2

Cooking Time: xx

Ingredients:

- 100g pasta
- 50g basil leaves
- 6 artichoke hearts
- 2 tbsp pumpkin seeds
- 2 tbsp lemon juice
- 1 clove garlic
- ½ tsp white miso paste
- 1 can chickpeas
- 1 tsp olive oil

Directions:

1. Place the chickpeas in the air fryer and cook at 200ºC for 12 minutes
2. Cook the pasta according to packet instructions
3. Add the remaining ingredients to a food processor and blend
4. Add the pasta to a bowl and spoon over the pesto mix
5. Serve and top with roasted chickpeas

Crispy Potato Peels

Servings: 1

Cooking Time: xx

Ingredients:

- Peels from 4 potatoes
- Cooking spray
- Salt to season

Directions:

1. Heat the air fryer to 200ºC
2. Place the peels in the air fryer spray with oil and sprinkle with salt
3. Cook for about 6-8 minutes until crispy

Tomato And Herb Tofu

Servings: 4

Cooking Time: 10 Minutes

Ingredients:

- 1 x 400 g / 14 oz block firm tofu
- 1 tbsp soy sauce
- 2 tbsp tomato paste
- 1 tsp dried oregano
- 1 tsp dried basil
- 1 tsp garlic powder

Directions:

1. Remove the tofu from the packaging and place on a sheet of kitchen roll. Place another sheet of kitchen roll on top of the tofu and place a plate on top of it.
2. Use something heavy to press the plate down on top of the tofu. Leave for 10 minutes to press the water out of the tofu.
3. Remove the paper towels from the tofu and chop them into even slices that are around ½ cm thick.
4. Preheat the air fryer to 180 °C / 350 °F. Remove the mesh basket from the air fryer machine and line with parchment paper.
5. Place the tofu slices on a lined baking sheet.
6. In a bowl, mix the soy sauce, tomato paste, dried oregano, dried basil, and garlic powder until fully combined.
7. Spread the mixture evenly over the tofu slices. Place the tofu slices on the baking sheet in the lined air fryer basket and cook for 10 minutes until the tofu is firm and crispy.
8. Serve the tofu slices with a side of rice or noodles and some hot vegetables.

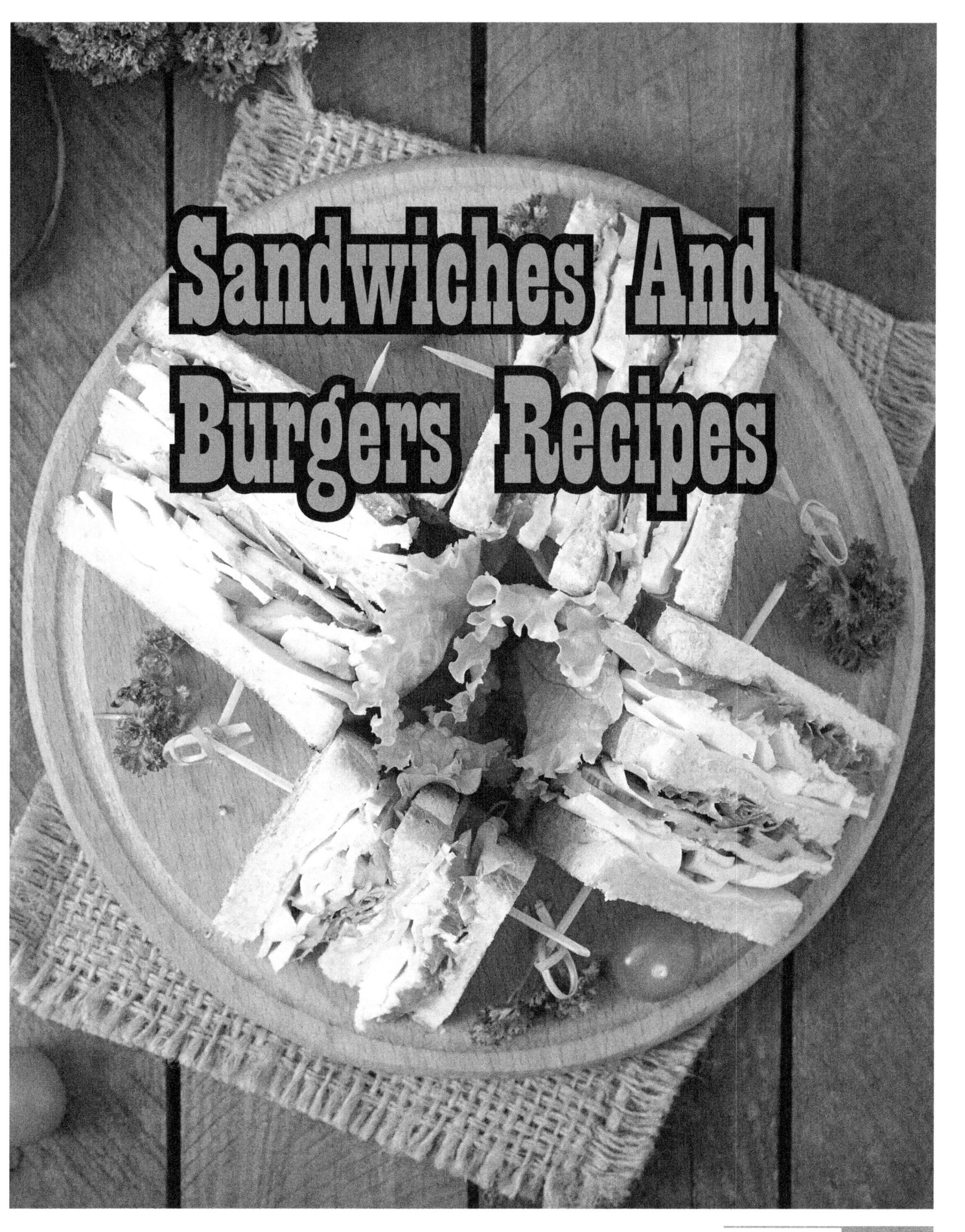

Sandwiches And Burgers Recipes

Sandwiches And Burgers Recipes

Inside Out Cheeseburgers

Servings: 2

Cooking Time: 20 Minutes

Ingredients:

- 340 grams lean ground beef
- 3 tablespoons minced onion
- 4 teaspoons ketchup
- 2 teaspoons yellow mustard
- Salt and freshly ground black pepper
- 4 slices of Cheddar cheese, broken into smaller pieces
- 8 hamburger dill pickle chips

Directions:

1. Combine the ground beef, minced onion, ketchup, mustard, salt, and pepper in a large bowl. Mix well to thoroughly combine the ingredients. Divide the meat into four equal portions.
2. To make the stuffed burgers, flatten each portion of meat into a thin patty. Place 4 pickle chips and half of the cheese onto the center of two of the patties, leaving a rim around the edge of the patty exposed. Place the remaining two patties on top of the first and press the meat together firmly, sealing the edges tightly. With the burgers on a flat surface, press the sides of the burger with the palm of your hand to create a straight edge. This will help keep the stuffing inside the burger while it cooks.
3. Preheat the air fryer to 190°C (370°F).
4. Place the burgers inside the air fryer basket and air-fry for 20 minutes, flipping the burgers over halfway through the cooking time.
5. Serve the cheeseburgers on buns with lettuce and tomato.

Mexican Cheeseburgers

Servings: 4

Cooking Time: 22 Minutes

Ingredients:

- 567 grams ground beef
- 60 grams finely chopped onion
- 60 grams crushed yellow corn tortilla chips
- 35 grams (1.25-ounce) packet taco seasoning
- 60 grams canned diced green chilies
- 1 egg, lightly beaten
- 113 grams pepper jack cheese, grated
- 4 (12-inch) flour tortillas
- shredded lettuce, sour cream, guacamole, salsa (for topping)

Directions:

1. Combine the ground beef, minced onion, crushed tortilla chips, taco seasoning, green chilies, and egg in a large bowl. Mix thoroughly until combined – your hands are good tools for this. Divide the meat into four equal portions and shape each portion into an oval-shaped burger.
2. Preheat the air fryer to 188°C (370°F).
3. Air-fry the burgers for 18 minutes, turning them over halfway through the cooking time. Divide the cheese between the burgers, lower fryer to 171°C (340°F), and air-fry for an additional 4 minutes to melt the cheese. (This will give you a burger that is medium-well. If you prefer your cheeseburger medium-rare, shorten the cooking time to about 15 minutes and then add the cheese and proceed with the recipe.)
4. While the burgers are cooking, warm the tortillas wrapped in aluminum foil in a 176°C (350°F) oven or in a skillet with a little oil over medium-high heat for a couple of minutes. Keep the tortillas warm until the burgers are ready.
5. To assemble the burgers, spread sour cream over three-quarters of the tortillas and top each with some shredded lettuce and salsa. Place the Mexican cheeseburgers on the lettuce and top with guacamole. Fold the tortillas around the burger, starting with the bottom and then folding the sides in over the top. (A little sour cream can help hold the seam of the tortilla together.) Serve immediately.

Provolone Stuffed Meatballs

Servings: 4

Cooking Time: 12 Minutes

Ingredients:

- 15 milliliters olive oil
- 1 small onion, very finely chopped
- 1 to 2 cloves garlic, minced
- 340 grams ground beef
- 340 grams ground pork
- 180 milliliters breadcrumbs
- 60 grams grated Parmesan cheese
- 60 milliliters finely chopped fresh parsley (or 15 milliliters dried parsley)
- 2.5 milliliters dried oregano
- 7.5 milliliters salt
- freshly ground black pepper
- 2 eggs, lightly beaten
- 142 grams sharp or aged provolone cheese, cut into 2.5-centimeter (1-inch) cubes

Directions:

1. Preheat a skillet over medium-high heat. Add the oil and cook the onion and garlic until tender, but not browned.
2. Transfer the onion and garlic to a large bowl and add the beef, pork, breadcrumbs, Parmesan cheese, parsley, oregano, salt, pepper, and eggs. Mix well until all the ingredients are combined.
3. Divide the mixture into 12 evenly sized balls. Make one meatball at a time by pressing a hole in the meatball mixture with your finger and pushing a piece of provolone cheese into the hole. Mold the meat back into a ball, enclosing the cheese.
4. Preheat the air fryer to 193°C (380°F).
5. Working in two batches, transfer six of the meatballs to the air fryer basket and air-fry for 12 minutes, shaking the basket and turning the meatballs a couple of times during the cooking process. Repeat with the remaining six meatballs. You can pop the first batch of meatballs into the air fryer for the last two minutes of cooking to re-heat them. Serve warm.

Black Bean Veggie Burgers

Servings: 3

Cooking Time: 10 Minutes

Ingredients:

- 225g Drained and rinsed canned black beans
- 40g Pecan pieces
- 40g Rolled oats (not quick-cooking or steel-cut; gluten-free, if needed)
- 30ml Pasteurized egg substitute (or 1 small egg), such as Egg Beaters (gluten-free, if needed)
- 10ml Red ketchup-like chili sauce, such as Heinz
- 2.5ml Ground cumin
- 2.5ml Dried oregano
- 2.5ml Table salt
- 2.5ml Ground black pepper
- Olive oil
- Olive oil spray

Directions:

1. Preheat the air fryer to 200°C (400°F).
2. Put the beans, pecans, oats, egg substitute or egg, chili sauce, cumin, oregano, salt, and pepper in a food processor. Cover and process to a coarse paste that will hold its shape like sugar-cookie dough, adding olive oil in 5ml increments to get the mixture to blend smoothly. The amount of olive oil is actually dependent on the internal moisture content of the beans and the oats. Figure on about 15ml (three 5ml additions) for the smaller batch, with proportional increases for the other batches. A little too much olive oil can't hurt, but a dry paste will fall apart as it cooks and a far-too-wet paste will stick to the basket.
3. Scrape down and remove the blade. Using clean, wet hands, form the paste into two 10cm patties for the small batch, three 10cm patties for the medium, or four 10cm patties for the large batch, setting them one by one on a cutting board.
4. Generously coat both sides of the patties with olive oil spray.
5. Set them in the basket in one layer. Air-fry undisturbed for 10 minutes, or until lightly browned and crisp at the edges.
6. Use a nonstick-safe spatula, and perhaps a flatware fork for balance, to transfer the burgers to a wire rack.Cool for 5 minutes before serving.

Inside-out Cheeseburgers

Servings: 3

Cooking Time: 9-11 Minutes

Ingredients:

- 510 grams lean ground beef (90% lean)
- ¾ teaspoon dried oregano
- ¾ teaspoon table salt
- ¾ teaspoon ground black pepper
- ¼ teaspoon garlic powder
- 45 grams (about 40g) shredded Cheddar, Swiss, or other semi-firm cheese, or a purchased blend of shredded cheeses
- 3 hamburger buns (gluten-free, if a concern), split open

Directions:

1. Preheat the air fryer to 190°C (375°F).
2. Gently mix the ground beef, oregano, salt, pepper, and garlic powder in a bowl until well combined without turning the mixture to mush. Form it into two 6-inch patties for the small batch, three for the medium, or four for the large.
3. Place 2 tablespoons of the shredded cheese in the center of each patty. With clean hands, fold the sides of the patty up to cover the cheese, then pick it up and roll it gently into a ball to seal the cheese inside. Gently press it back into a 5-inch burger without letting any cheese squish out. Continue filling and preparing more burgers, as needed.
4. Place the burgers in the basket in one layer and air-fry undisturbed for 8 minutes for medium or 10 minutes for well-done. (An instant-read meat thermometer won't work for these burgers because it will hit the mostly melted cheese inside and offer a hotter temperature than the surrounding meat.)
5. Use a nonstick-safe spatula, and perhaps a flatware fork for balance, to transfer the burgers to a cutting board. Set the buns cut side down in the basket in one layer (working in batches as necessary) and air-fry undisturbed for 1 minute, to toast a bit and warm up. Cool the burgers a few minutes more, then serve them warm in the buns.

Salmon Burgers

Servings: 3

Cooking Time: 8 Minutes

Ingredients:

- 510 grams Skinless salmon fillet, preferably fattier Atlantic salmon
- 22.5 milliliters Minced chives or the green part of a scallion
- 120 milliliters Plain panko bread crumbs (gluten-free, if a concern)
- 7.5 milliliters Dijon mustard (gluten-free, if a concern)
- 7.5 milliliters Drained and rinsed capers, minced
- 7.5 milliliters Lemon juice
- 1.25 milliliters Table salt
- 1.25 milliliters Ground black pepper
- Vegetable oil spray

Directions:

1. Preheat the air fryer to 190°C (375°F).
2. Cut the salmon into pieces that will fit in a food processor. Cover and pulse until coarsely chopped. Add the chives and pulse to combine, until the fish is ground but not a paste. Scrape down and remove the blade. Scrape the salmon mixture into a bowl. Add the bread crumbs, mustard, capers, lemon juice, salt, and pepper. Stir gently until well combined.
3. Use clean and dry hands to form the mixture into two 5-inch patties for a small batch, three 5-inch patties for a medium batch, or four 5-inch patties for a large one.
4. Coat both sides of each patty with vegetable oil spray. Set them in the basket in one layer and air-fry undisturbed for 8 minutes, or until browned and an instant-read meat thermometer inserted into the center of a burger registers 63°C (145°F).
5. Use a nonstick-safe spatula, and perhaps a flatware fork for balance, to transfer the burgers to a wire rack. Cool for 2 or 3 minutes before serving.

Dijon Thyme Burgers

Servings: 3

Cooking Time: 18 Minutes

Ingredients:

- 450 grams lean ground beef
- 30 grams panko breadcrumbs
- 25 grams finely chopped onion
- 45 milliliters Dijon mustard
- 15 milliliters chopped fresh thyme
- 20 milliliters Worcestershire sauce
- 5 grams salt
- Freshly ground black pepper
- Topping (optional):
- 30 milliliters Dijon mustard
- 15 grams dark brown sugar
- 5 milliliters Worcestershire sauce
- 115 grams sliced Swiss cheese, optional

Directions:

1. Combine all the burger ingredients together in a large bowl and mix well. Divide the meat into 4 equal portions and then form the burgers, being careful not to over-handle the meat. One good way to do this is to throw the meat back and forth from one hand to another, packing the meat each time you catch it. Flatten the balls into patties, making an indentation in the center of each patty with your thumb (this will help it stay flat as it cooks) and flattening the sides of the burgers so that they will fit nicely into the air fryer basket.
2. Preheat the air fryer to 190°C (370°F).
3. If you don't have room for all four burgers, air-fry two or three burgers at a time for 8 minutes. Flip the burgers over and air-fry for another 6 minutes.
4. While the burgers are cooking, combine the Dijon mustard, dark brown sugar, and Worcestershire sauce in a small bowl and mix well. This optional topping for the burgers adds a boost of flavor at the end. Spread the Dijon topping evenly on each burger. If you cooked the burgers in batches, return the first batch to the cooker at this time – it's ok to place the fourth burger on top of the others in the center of the basket. Air-fry the burgers for another 3 minutes.
5. Finally, if desired, top each burger with a slice of Swiss cheese. Lower the air fryer temperature to 165°C (330°F) and air-fry for another minute to melt the cheese. Serve the burgers on toasted brioche buns, dressed the way you like them.

Chicken Apple Brie Melt

Servings: 3

Cooking Time: 13 Minutes

Ingredients:

- 3 boneless skinless chicken breasts (approximately 140-170g each)
- Vegetable oil spray
- 7.5ml Dried herbes de Provence
- 85g Brie, rind removed, thinly sliced
- 6 Thin cored apple slices
- 3 French rolls (gluten-free, if needed)
- 30ml Dijon mustard (gluten-free, if needed)

Directions:

1. Preheat the air fryer to 190°C (375°F).
2. Lightly coat all sides of the chicken breasts with vegetable oil spray. Sprinkle the breasts evenly with the herbes de Provence.
3. When the air fryer is at temperature, place the breasts in the basket and air-fry undisturbed for 10 minutes.
4. Top the chicken breasts with the apple slices, then the cheese. Air-fry undisturbed for 2 minutes, or until the cheese is melty and bubbling.
5. Use a nonstick-safe spatula and kitchen tongs, for balance, to transfer the breasts to a cutting board. Set the rolls in the basket and air-fry for 1 minute to warm through. (Putting them in the machine without splitting them keeps the insides very soft while the outside gets a little crunchy.)
6. Transfer the rolls to the cutting board. Split them open lengthwise, then spread 5ml of mustard on each cut side. Set a prepared chicken breast on the bottom of a roll and close with its top, repeating as necessary to make additional sandwiches. Serve warm.

Turkey Burgers

Servings: 3

Cooking Time: 23 Minutes

Ingredients:

- 500 grams Ground turkey
- 90 grams Frozen chopped spinach, thawed and squeezed dry
- 45 grams Plain panko bread crumbs (ensure they are gluten-free if needed)
- 15 grams Dijon mustard (ensure it's gluten-free if needed)
- 7.5 grams Minced garlic
- 3/4 teaspoon Table salt
- 3/4 teaspoon Ground black pepper
- Olive oil spray
- 3 Kaiser rolls (ensure they are gluten-free if needed), split open

Directions:

1. Preheat your air fryer to 190°C (375°F).
2. In a large bowl, gently combine the ground turkey, thawed and squeezed dry chopped spinach, panko bread crumbs, Dijon mustard, minced garlic, salt, and black pepper. Try to maintain some of the ground turkey's texture. Form the mixture into two 17 cm (5-inch) wide patties for a small batch, three patties for a medium batch, or four patties for a large batch.
3. Coat each side of the patties with olive oil spray.
4. Place the patties in the air fryer basket in a single layer. Air-fry without disturbing for 20 minutes or until an instant-read meat thermometer inserted into the center of a burger registers 74°C (165°F). If your air fryer is set to 180°C (360°F), you may need to add an additional 2 minutes to the cooking time.
5. Use a spatula that is safe for nonstick surfaces, and perhaps a flatware fork for balance, to transfer the burgers to a cutting board.
6. Place the split Kaiser rolls cut side down in the air fryer basket in a single layer (you may need to work in batches) and air-fry for 1 minute to lightly toast and warm them.
7. Serve the turkey burgers warm in the buns.

Perfect Burgers

Servings: 3

Cooking Time: 13 Minutes

Ingredients:

- 530 grams 90% lean ground beef
- 22.5 milliliters Worcestershire sauce (gluten-free, if a concern)
- 2.5 grams Ground black pepper
- 3 Hamburger buns (gluten-free if a concern), split open

Directions:

1. Preheat the air fryer to 190°C (375°F).
2. Gently mix the ground beef, Worcestershire sauce, and pepper in a bowl until well combined but preserving as much of the meat's fibers as possible. Divide this mixture into two 17 cm (5-inch) patties for the small batch, three 12.7 cm (5-inch) patties for the medium, or four 12.7 cm (5-inch) patties for the large. Make a thumbprint indentation in the center of each patty, about halfway through the meat.
3. Set the patties in the basket in one layer with some space between them. Air-fry undisturbed for 10 minutes, or until an instant-read meat thermometer inserted into the center of a burger registers 71°C (160°F) (a medium-well burger). You may need to add 2 minutes of cooking time if the air fryer is at 182°C (360°F).
4. Use a nonstick-safe spatula, and perhaps a flatware fork for balance, to transfer the burgers to a cutting board. Set the buns cut side down in the basket in one layer (working in batches as necessary) and air-fry undisturbed for 1 minute, to toast a bit and warm up. Serve the burgers in the warm buns.

Air Fryer Cookbook

Chicken Spiedies

Servings: 3

Cooking Time: 12 Minutes

Ingredients:

- 567 grams boneless, skinless chicken thighs, trimmed of any fat blobs and cut into 5-cm pieces
- 45 ml red wine vinegar
- 30 ml olive oil
- 30 ml minced fresh mint leaves
- 30 ml minced fresh parsley leaves
- 30 ml minced fresh dill fronds
- 2.25 ml fennel seeds
- 2.25 ml table salt
- Up to 1.25 ml red pepper flakes
- 3 long soft rolls, such as hero, hoagie, or Italian sub rolls (gluten-free, if a concern), split open lengthwise
- 67.5 ml regular or low-fat mayonnaise (not fat-free; gluten-free, if a concern)
- 22.5 ml distilled white vinegar
- 7.5 ml ground black pepper

Directions:

1. Mix the chicken, vinegar, oil, mint, parsley, dill, fennel seeds, salt, and red pepper flakes in a zip-closed plastic bag. Seal, gently massage the marinade ingredients into the meat, and refrigerate for at least 2 hours or up to 6 hours. (Longer than that and the meat can turn rubbery.)
2. Set the plastic bag out on the counter (to make the contents a little less frigid). Preheat the air fryer to 200°C (400°F).
3. When the machine is at temperature, use kitchen tongs to set the chicken thighs in the basket (discard any remaining marinade) and air-fry undisturbed for 6 minutes. Turn the thighs over and continue air-frying undisturbed for 6 minutes more, until well browned, cooked through, and even a little crunchy.
4. Dump the contents of the basket onto a wire rack and cool for 2 or 3 minutes. Divide the chicken evenly between the rolls.
5. Whisk the mayonnaise, vinegar, and black pepper in a small bowl until smooth. Drizzle this sauce over the chicken pieces in the rolls.

Sausage And Pepper Subs

Servings: 3

Cooking Time: 11 Minutes

Ingredients:

- 3 Sweet Italian sausages (approximately 255 grams total) (ensure they are gluten-free if needed)
- 1½ Medium red or green bell peppers, deseeded and cut into 1.25 cm wide strips
- 1 medium Yellow or white onion, peeled, halved, and thinly sliced into half-moons
- 3 Long soft rolls, like sub rolls or baguettes (ensure they are gluten-free if needed), split open lengthwise
- Balsamic vinegar, for garnish
- Fresh basil leaves, for garnish
- Instructions:
- Preheat your air fryer to 200°C (400°F).
- Once the air fryer reaches the desired temperature, place the sausage links in the basket in a single layer. Air-fry without disturbance for 5 minutes.
- Add the pepper strips and onions to the air fryer. Continue air-frying, tossing and rearranging them every minute for 5 minutes, or until the sausages are browned and an instant-read meat thermometer inserted into one of the sausages registers 71°C (160°F).
- Use a spatula that is safe for nonstick surfaces and kitchen tongs to transfer the sausages and vegetables to a cutting board.
- Place the rolls cut side down in the air fryer basket in a single layer (you may need to work in batches) and air-fry for 1 minute without disturbance to lightly toast and warm them.
- Place one sausage along with some pepper strips and onions into each warmed roll. Drizzle a bit of balsamic vinegar over the sandwich fillings and garnish with fresh basil leaves.

White Bean Veggie Burgers

Servings: 3

Cooking Time: 13 Minutes

Ingredients:

- 300 grams Drained and rinsed canned white beans
- 45 grams Rolled oats (not quick-cooking or steel-cut; ensure they are gluten-free if needed)
- 45 grams Chopped walnuts
- 10 milliliters Olive oil
- 10 milliliters Lemon juice
- 7.5 milliliters Dijon mustard (ensure it's gluten-free if needed)
- 3.75 milliliters Dried sage leaves
- 1.25 milliliters Table salt
- Olive oil spray
- 3 Whole-wheat buns or gluten-free whole-grain buns (if needed), split open

Directions:

1. Preheat your air fryer to 200°C (400°F).
2. In a food processor, combine the drained and rinsed canned white beans, rolled oats, chopped walnuts, olive oil, lemon juice, Dijon mustard, dried sage leaves, and table salt. Process until you achieve a coarse paste with a consistency similar to wet sugar-cookie dough. Make sure to stop the machine and scrape down the sides of the canister at least once during processing.
3. Scrape down and remove the blade from the food processor. With clean, wet hands, shape the bean paste into two 10.16 cm (4-inch) patties for a small batch, three patties for a medium batch, or four patties for a large batch. Generously coat each patty on both sides with olive oil spray.
4. Place the patties in the air fryer basket, leaving some space between them. Air-fry without disturbance for 12 minutes or until the patties are lightly browned and crisp at the edges. The tops of the burgers should feel firm to the touch.
5. Use a spatula that is safe for nonstick surfaces, and perhaps a flatware fork for balance, to transfer the burgers to a cutting board.
6. Place the split buns cut side down in the air fryer basket in a single layer (you may need to work in batches) and air-fry for 1 minute to lightly toast and warm them.
7. Serve the veggie burgers warm in the buns.

Chicken Saltimbocca Sandwiches

Servings: 3

Cooking Time: 11 Minutes

Ingredients:

- 3 boneless, skinless chicken breasts (about 150-180g each)
- 6 thin prosciutto slices
- 6 provolone cheese slices
- 3 long soft rolls, such as hero, hoagie, or Italian sub rolls (gluten-free, if needed), split open lengthwise
- 3 tablespoons pesto, purchased or homemade (see the headnote)

Directions:

1. Preheat the air fryer to 200°C (400°F).
2. Wrap each chicken breast with 2 prosciutto slices, spiraling the prosciutto around the breast and overlapping the slices a bit to cover the breast. The prosciutto will stick to the chicken more readily than bacon does.
3. When the machine is at temperature, set the wrapped chicken breasts in the basket and air-fry undisturbed for 10 minutes, or until the prosciutto is frizzled and the chicken is cooked through.
4. Overlap 2 cheese slices on each breast. Air-fry undisturbed for 1 minute, or until melted. Take the basket out of the machine.
5. Smear the insides of the rolls with the pesto, then use kitchen tongs to put a wrapped and cheesy chicken breast in each roll.

Chicken Gyros

Servings: 4

Cooking Time: 14 Minutes

Ingredients:

- 4 boneless skinless chicken thighs (approximately 110-140g each), trimmed of any fat blobs
- 30ml Lemon juice
- 30ml Red wine vinegar
- 30ml Olive oil
- 10g Dried oregano
- 10g Minced garlic
- 5g Table salt
- 5g Ground black pepper
- 4 Pita pockets (gluten-free, if needed)
- 120g Chopped tomatoes
- 120ml Bottled regular, low-fat, or fat-free ranch dressing (gluten-free, if needed)

Directions:

1. Mix the thighs, lemon juice, vinegar, oil, oregano, garlic, salt, and pepper in a zip-closed bag. Seal the bag, gently massage the marinade into the meat through the plastic, and refrigerate for at least 2 hours or up to 6 hours. (Marinating longer can result in rubbery meat.)
2. Set the plastic bag out on the counter (to make the contents a little less cold). Preheat the air fryer to 190°C (375°F).
3. When the air fryer reaches temperature, use kitchen tongs to place the thighs in the basket in a single layer. Discard the marinade. Air-fry the chicken thighs undisturbed for 12 minutes, or until browned and an instant-read meat thermometer inserted into the thickest part of one thigh registers 74°C (165°F). You may need to air-fry the chicken for an additional 2 minutes if the air fryer's temperature is at 180°C (360°F).
4. Use kitchen tongs to transfer the thighs to a cutting board. Let them cool for 5 minutes, then place one thigh in each of the pita pockets. Top each with 30g chopped tomatoes and 30ml dressing. Serve warm.

Eggplant Parmesan Subs

Servings: 2

Cooking Time: 13 Minutes

Ingredients:

- 4 Peeled eggplant slices (about 1.25 cm thick and 7.5 cm in diameter)
- Olive oil spray
- 2 tablespoons plus 2 teaspoons Jarred pizza sauce, any variety except creamy
- 25 grams Finely grated Parmesan cheese
- 2 Small, long soft rolls, such as hero, hoagie, or Italian sub rolls (gluten-free, if a concern), split open lengthwise

Directions:

1. Preheat the air fryer to 175°C (350°F).
2. When the machine is at temperature, coat both sides of the eggplant slices with olive oil spray. Set them in the basket in one layer and air-fry undisturbed for 10 minutes, until lightly browned and softened.
3. Increase the machine's temperature to 190°C (375°F) (or 190°C, if that's the closest setting—unless the machine is already at 180°C, in which case leave it alone). Top each eggplant slice with 2 teaspoons pizza sauce, then 1 tablespoon cheese. Air-fry undisturbed for 2 minutes, or until the cheese has melted.
4. Use a nonstick-safe spatula, and perhaps a flatware fork for balance, to transfer the eggplant slices cheese side up to a cutting board. Set the roll(s) cut side down in the basket in one layer (working in batches as necessary) and air-fry undisturbed for 1 minute, to toast the rolls a bit and warm them up. Set 2 eggplant slices in each warm roll.

Reuben Sandwiches

Servings: 2

Cooking Time: 11 Minutes

Ingredients:

- 227 grams Sliced deli corned beef
- 20 milliliters Regular or low-fat mayonnaise (not fat-free)
- 4 Rye bread slices
- 30 milliliters Russian dressing
- 120 milliliters Purchased sauerkraut, squeezed by the handful over the sink to get rid of excess moisture
- 56 grams (2 to 4 slices) Swiss cheese slices (optional)

Directions:

1. Set the corned beef in the basket, slip the basket into the air fryer, and heat it to 204°C (400°F). Air-fry undisturbed for 3 minutes from the time the basket is put in the machine, just to warm up the meat.
2. Use kitchen tongs to transfer the corned beef to a cutting board. Spread 5 milliliters (1 teaspoon) mayonnaise on one side of each slice of rye bread, rubbing the mayonnaise into the bread with a small flatware knife.
3. Place the bread slices mayonnaise side down on a cutting board. Spread the Russian dressing over the "dry" side of each slice. For one sandwich, top one slice of bread with the corned beef, sauerkraut, and cheese (if using). For two sandwiches, top two slices of bread each with half of the corned beef, sauerkraut, and cheese (if using). Close the sandwiches with the remaining bread, setting it mayonnaise side up on top.
4. Set the sandwich(es) in the basket and air-fry undisturbed for 8 minutes, or until browned and crunchy.
5. Use a nonstick-safe spatula, and perhaps a flatware fork for balance, to transfer the sandwich(es) to a cutting board. Cool for 2 or 3 minutes before slicing in half and serving.

Chili Cheese Dogs

Servings: 3

Cooking Time: 12 Minutes

Ingredients:

- 340 grams lean ground beef
- 22.5 ml chile powder
- 240 ml plus 30 ml jarred sofrito
- 3 Hot dogs (gluten-free, if a concern)
- 3 Hot dog buns (gluten-free, if a concern), split open lengthwise
- 45 ml finely chopped scallion
- 270 ml (a little more than 57 grams) Shredded Cheddar cheese

Directions:

1. Crumble the ground beef into a medium or large saucepan set over medium heat. Brown well, stirring often to break up the clumps. Add the chile powder and cook for 30 seconds, stirring the whole time. Stir in the sofrito and bring to a simmer. Reduce the heat to low and simmer, stirring occasionally, for 5 minutes. Keep warm.
2. Preheat the air fryer to 200°C (400°F).
3. When the machine is at temperature, put the hot dogs in the basket and air-fry undisturbed for 10 minutes, or until the hot dogs are bubbling and blistered, even a little crisp.
4. Use kitchen tongs to put the hot dogs in the buns. Top each with 150 ml of the ground beef mixture, 15 ml of the minced scallion, and 90 ml of the cheese. (The scallion should go under the cheese so it superheats and wilts a bit.) Set the filled hot dog buns in the basket and air-fry undisturbed for 2 minutes, or until the cheese has melted.
5. Remove the basket from the machine. Cool the chili cheese dogs in the basket for 5 minutes before serving.

Air Fryer Cookbook

Best-ever Roast Beef Sandwiches

Servings: 6

Cooking Time: 30-50 Minutes

Ingredients:

- 12.5ml Olive oil
- 7.5ml Dried oregano
- 7.5ml Dried thyme
- 7.5ml Onion powder
- 7.5ml Table salt
- 7.5ml Ground black pepper
- 1.4kg Beef eye of round
- 6 Round soft rolls, such as Kaiser rolls or hamburger buns (gluten-free, if needed), split open lengthwise
- 180ml Regular, low-fat, or fat-free mayonnaise (gluten-free, if needed)
- 6 Romaine lettuce leaves, rinsed
- 6 Round tomato slices (6mm thick)

Directions:

1. Preheat the air fryer to 175°C (350°F).
2. Mix the olive oil, dried oregano, dried thyme, onion powder, salt, and black pepper in a small bowl. Spread this mixture all over the eye of round.
3. When the air fryer is at temperature, place the beef in the basket and air-fry for 30 to 50 minutes (the range depends on the size of the cut), turning the meat twice. Use an instant-read meat thermometer inserted into the thickest piece of meat to register 54°C for rare, 60°C for medium, or 65°C for well-done.
4. Use kitchen tongs to transfer the beef to a cutting board. Allow it to cool for 10 minutes.
5. If serving immediately, carve the beef into 3mm thick slices. Spread each roll with 30ml of mayonnaise and divide the beef slices between the rolls. Top with a lettuce leaf and a tomato slice and serve.
6. Alternatively, place the beef in a container, cover, and refrigerate for up to 3 days to make cold roast beef sandwiches anytime.

Asian Glazed Meatballs

Servings: 4

Cooking Time: 10 Minutes

Ingredients:

- 1 large shallot, finely chopped
- 2 cloves garlic, minced
- 1 tablespoon grated fresh ginger
- 2 teaspoons fresh thyme, finely chopped
- 225g brown mushrooms, very finely chopped (a food processor works well here)
- 30ml soy sauce
- Freshly ground black pepper
- 450g ground beef
- 225g ground pork
- 3 egg yolks
- 240ml Thai sweet chili sauce (spring roll sauce)
- 60g toasted sesame seeds
- 2 scallions, sliced

Directions:

1. Combine the shallot, garlic, ginger, thyme, mushrooms, soy sauce, freshly ground black pepper, ground beef and pork, and egg yolks in a bowl. Mix the ingredients together. Gently shape the mixture into 24 balls, about the size of a golf ball.
2. Preheat the air fryer to 190°C (380°F).
3. Working in batches, air-fry the meatballs for 8 minutes, turning the meatballs over halfway through the cooking time.
4. Drizzle some of the Thai sweet chili sauce on top of each meatball and return the basket to the air fryer. Air-fry for another 2 minutes. Reserve the remaining Thai sweet chili sauce for serving.
5. As soon as the meatballs are done, sprinkle them with toasted sesame seeds and transfer them to a serving platter.
6. Scatter the sliced scallions around and serve the meatballs warm.

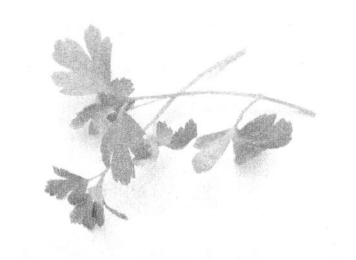

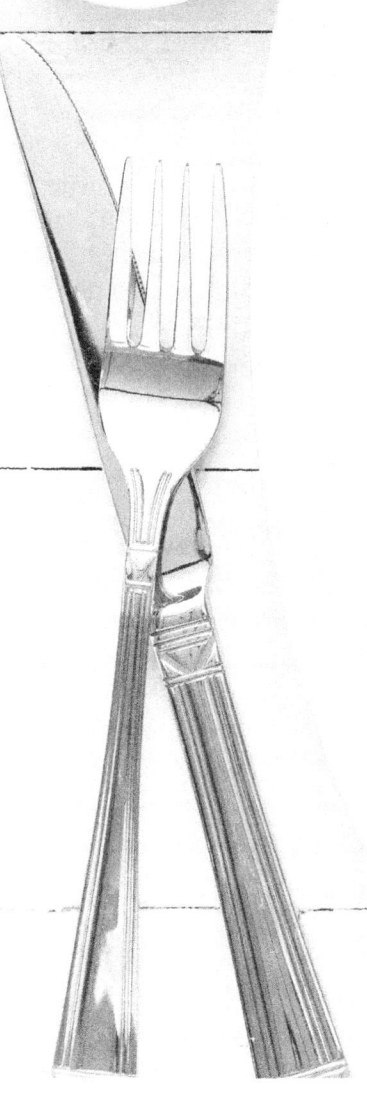

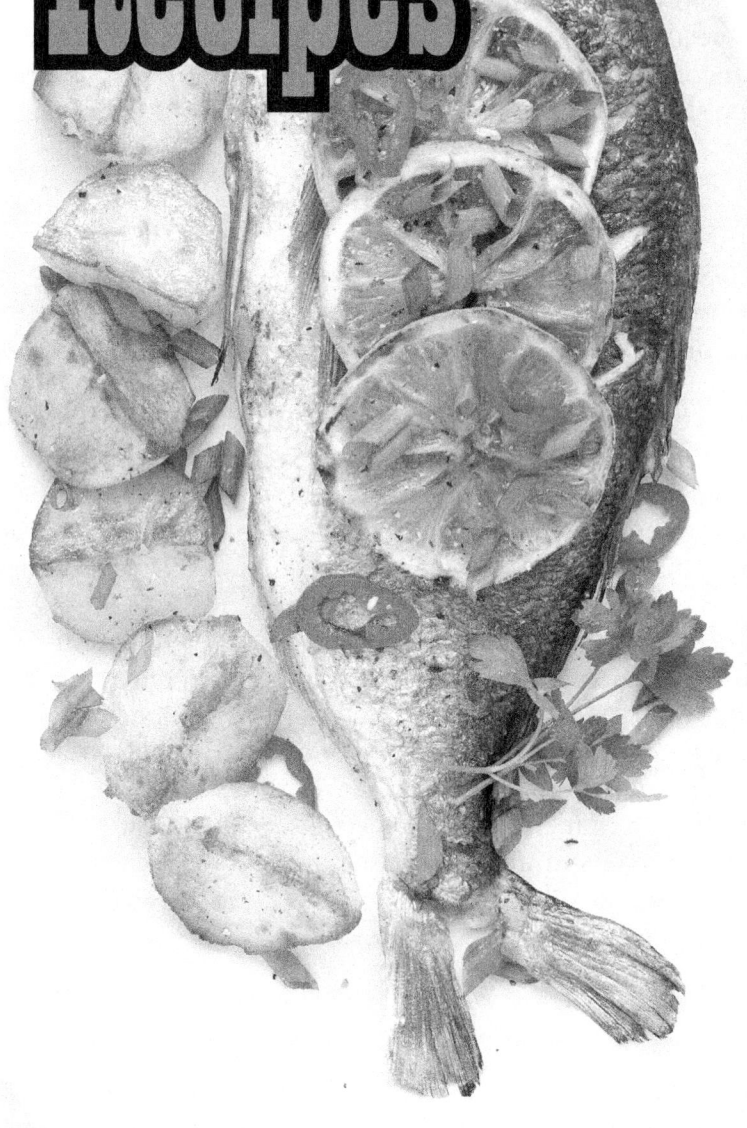

Fish And Seafood Recipes

Fish And Seafood Recipes

Pecan-orange Crusted Striped Bass

Servings: 2

Cooking Time: 9 Minutes

Ingredients:

- Flour, for dredging*
- 2 egg whites, lightly beaten
- 100 grams pecans, chopped
- 1 teaspoon finely chopped orange zest, plus more for garnish
- ½ teaspoon salt
- 2 (170-gram) fillets striped bass
- Salt and freshly ground black pepper
- Vegetable or olive oil, in a spray bottle
- Orange Cream Sauce (Optional)
- 120 ml fresh orange juice
- 60 ml heavy cream
- 1 sprig fresh thyme

Directions:

1. Set up a dredging station with three shallow dishes. Place the flour in one shallow dish. Place the beaten egg whites in a second shallow dish. Finally, combine the chopped pecans, orange zest, and salt in a third shallow dish.
2. Coat the fish fillets one at a time. First, season with salt and freshly ground black pepper. Then, coat each fillet in flour. Shake off any excess flour and then dip the fish into the egg white. Let the excess egg drip off, and then immediately press the fish into the pecan-orange mixture. Set the crusted fish fillets aside.
3. Preheat the air fryer to 200°C.
4. Spray the crusted fish with oil and then transfer the fillets to the air fryer basket. Air-fry for 9 minutes at 200°C, flipping the fish over halfway through the cooking time. The nuts on top should be nice and toasty, and the fish should feel firm to the touch.
5. If you'd like to make a sauce to go with the fish while it cooks, combine the freshly squeezed orange juice, heavy cream, and sprig of thyme in a small saucepan. Simmer on the stovetop for 5 minutes and then set aside.
6. Remove the fish from the air fryer and serve over a bed of salad, like the one below. Then add a sprinkling of orange zest and a spoonful of the orange cream sauce over the top if desired.

Maple-crusted Salmon

Servings: 2

Cooking Time: 8 Minutes

Ingredients:

- 340 grams salmon fillets
- 80 ml maple syrup
- 5 ml Worcestershire sauce
- 10 ml Dijon mustard or brown mustard
- 65 grams finely chopped walnuts
- 2.5 ml sea salt
- ½ lemon
- 15 ml chopped parsley, for garnish

Directions:

1. Place the salmon in a shallow baking dish. Top with maple syrup, Worcestershire sauce, and mustard. Refrigerate for 30 minutes.
2. Preheat the air fryer to 180°C.
3. Remove the salmon from the marinade and discard the marinade.
4. Place the chopped nuts on top of the salmon fillets, and sprinkle salt on top of the nuts. Place the salmon, skin side down, in the air fryer basket. Cook for 6 to 8 minutes or until the fish flakes in the center.
5. Remove the salmon and plate on a serving platter. Squeeze fresh lemon over the top of the salmon and top with chopped parsley. Serve immediately.

Cajun Flounder Fillets

Servings: 2

Cooking Time: 5 Minutes

Ingredients:

- 2 115g skinless flounder fillets
- 2 teaspoons peanut oil
- 1 teaspoon purchased or homemade Cajun dried seasoning blend (see note below)

Directions:

1. Preheat your air fryer to 200°C (400°F).
2. Drizzle the peanut oil over the flounder fillets, then gently rub the oil in with your clean, dry fingers.
3. Sprinkle the Cajun seasoning blend evenly over both sides of the fillets.
4. Once your air fryer reaches the desired temperature, place the flounder fillets in the basket. If you are cooking more than one fillet, ensure they do not touch, although they can be close together depending on the basket's size.
5. Air-fry the fillets undisturbed for 5 minutes or until they are lightly browned and cooked through.
6. Use a nonstick-safe spatula to transfer the cooked fillets to a serving platter or individual plates.
7. Serve your Cajun Flounder Fillets immediately.

Lime Bay Scallops

Servings: 4

Cooking Time: 10 Minutes

Ingredients:

- 30 milliliters butter, melted
- 1 lime, juiced
- 1.25 milliliters salt
- 450 grams bay scallops
- 30 milliliters chopped cilantro

Directions:

1. Preheat the air fryer to 180°C (350°F).
2. In a bowl, combine all the ingredients except for the cilantro.
3. Place the bay scallops in the air fryer basket.
4. Air fry for 5 minutes, tossing them once during cooking.
5. Serve the Lime Bay Scallops immediately, topped with chopped cilantro.

Caribbean Skewers

Servings: 4

Cooking Time: 25 Minutes

Ingredients:

- 680g large shrimp, peeled and deveined
- 1 can pineapple chunks, drained (reserve the liquid)
- 1 red bell pepper, chopped
- 3 scallions, chopped
- 15ml lemon juice
- 15ml olive oil
- 1/2 tsp jerk seasoning
- 1/8 tsp cayenne pepper
- 30ml cilantro, chopped

Directions:

1. Preheat your air fryer to 190°C (375°F).
2. Thread the large shrimp, pineapple chunks, red bell pepper, and scallions onto 8 bamboo skewers.
3. In a bowl, mix 45ml (3 tablespoons) of pineapple juice from the can with lemon juice, olive oil, jerk seasoning, and cayenne pepper.
4. Brush this mixture over the skewers, making sure to coat all sides.
5. Place 4 skewers in the air fryer basket and add a rack if necessary to accommodate the rest of the skewers on top.
6. Air fry for 6-9 minutes, and at around 4-5 minutes, rearrange the skewers to ensure even cooking.
7. Continue cooking until the shrimp curl and turn pink.
8. Sprinkle the freshly chopped cilantro over the cooked Caribbean Skewers.
9. Serve your delicious Caribbean Skewers immediately.

Beer-breaded Halibut Fish Tacos

Servings: 4

Cooking Time: 10 Minutes

Ingredients:

- 450g halibut, cut into 2.5cm strips
- 240ml light beer
- 1 jalapeño, minced and divided
- 1 clove garlic, minced
- 1g ground cumin
- 60g cornmeal
- 30g all-purpose flour
- 6.25g sea salt, divided
- 200g shredded cabbage
- 1 lime, juiced and divided
- 60ml Greek yogurt
- 60ml mayonnaise
- 200g grape tomatoes, quartered
- 30g chopped cilantro
- 60g chopped onion
- 1 egg, whisked
- 8 corn tortillas

Directions:

1. In a shallow baking dish, place the halibut, light beer, 1 teaspoon of minced jalapeño, minced garlic, and ground cumin. Cover and refrigerate for 30 minutes.
2. Meanwhile, in a medium bowl, mix together the cornmeal, flour, and ½ teaspoon of sea salt.
3. In a large bowl, combine the shredded cabbage, 1 tablespoon of lime juice, Greek yogurt, mayonnaise, and ½ teaspoon of sea salt.
4. In a small bowl, make the pico de gallo by mixing together the grape tomatoes, cilantro, chopped onion, ¼ teaspoon of sea salt, the remaining minced jalapeño, and the remaining lime juice.
5. Remove the fish from the refrigerator and discard the marinade. Dredge the fish in the whisked egg; then dredge the fish in the cornmeal flour mixture until all pieces of fish are breaded.
6. Preheat the air fryer to 175°C (350°F).
7. Place the fish in the air fryer basket and spray liberally with cooking spray. Cook for 6 minutes, flip and shake the fish, and cook for another 4 minutes.
8. While the fish is cooking, heat the tortillas in a heavy skillet for 1 to 2 minutes over high heat.
9. To assemble the tacos, place the battered fish on the heated tortillas and top with slaw and pico de gallo. Serve immediately.

Feta & Shrimp Pita

Servings: 4

Cooking Time: 15 Minutes

Ingredients:

- 450 grams peeled shrimp, deveined
- 30 ml olive oil
- 5 ml dried oregano
- 2.5 ml dried thyme
- 2.5 ml garlic powder
- 1.25 ml shallot powder
- 1.25 ml tarragon powder
- Salt and pepper to taste
- 4 whole-wheat pitas
- 115 grams feta cheese, crumbled
- 240 ml grated lettuce
- 1 tomato, diced
- 60 ml black olives, sliced
- 1 lemon

Directions:

1. Preheat the oven to 190°C (380°F).
2. In a bowl, mix the shrimp with olive oil, dried oregano, dried thyme, garlic powder, shallot powder, tarragon powder, salt, and pepper.
3. Arrange the shrimp in a single layer in the frying basket of the air fryer.
4. Bake for 6-8 minutes or until the shrimp are no longer pink and are cooked through.
5. While the shrimp are cooking, warm the whole-wheat pitas in the oven.
6. Divide the cooked shrimp into the warmed pitas and top with crumbled feta cheese, grated lettuce, diced tomato, sliced black olives, and a squeeze of lemon.
7. Serve your Feta & Shrimp Pita and enjoy!

Buttered Swordfish Steaks

Servings: 4

Cooking Time: 30 Minutes

Ingredients:

- 4 swordfish steaks
- 2 eggs, beaten
- 85g melted butter
- 120g breadcrumbs
- Black pepper to taste
- 1 tsp dried rosemary
- 1 tsp dried marjoram
- 1 lemon, cut into wedges

Directions:

1. Preheat your air fryer to 180°C (350°F).
2. In a bowl, thoroughly stir together the beaten eggs and melted butter.
3. In a separate bowl, combine the breadcrumbs, rosemary, marjoram, and black pepper.
4. Dip each swordfish steak into the beaten egg and butter mixture, ensuring they are well coated.
5. Coat the egg-covered steaks with the breadcrumb mixture, pressing it onto the fish to create a crust.
6. Place the coated swordfish steaks in the air fryer basket.
7. Air fry for 12-14 minutes, turning the steaks once during cooking to ensure they are cooked through and the crust is toasted and crispy.
8. Serve the Buttered Swordfish Steaks with lemon wedges.

Lemon & Herb Crusted Salmon

Servings: 4

Cooking Time: 20 Minutes

Ingredients:

- 80 grams crushed potato chips
- 4 skinless salmon fillets
- 45 milliliters honey mustard
- 2.5 milliliters lemon zest
- 2.5 milliliters dried thyme
- 2.5 milliliters dried basil
- 60 grams panko bread crumbs
- 30 milliliters olive oil

Directions:

1. Preheat the air fryer to 160°C (320°F).
2. Place the salmon fillets on a work surface.
3. In a small bowl, mix together the honey mustard, lemon zest, dried thyme, and dried basil. Spread this mixture evenly on top of the salmon fillets.
4. In a separate small bowl, combine the panko bread crumbs and crushed potato chips. Drizzle them with olive oil and mix well.
5. Place the salmon fillets in the air fryer basket.
6. Air fry until the salmon is cooked through and the topping is crispy and brown, which should take about 10 minutes.
7. Serve the Lemon & Herb Crusted Salmon hot and enjoy!

Garlic And Dill Salmon

Servings: 2

Cooking Time: 8 Minutes

Ingredients:

- 340 grams salmon fillets with skin
- 30 milliliters melted butter
- 15 milliliters extra-virgin olive oil
- 2 garlic cloves, minced
- 15 milliliters fresh dill
- 2.5 milliliters sea salt
- ½ lemon

Directions:

1. Pat the salmon dry with paper towels.
2. In a small bowl, combine the melted butter, olive oil, minced garlic, and fresh dill.
3. Sprinkle the top of the salmon with sea salt. Brush all sides of the salmon with the garlic and dill butter mixture.
4. Preheat the air fryer to 180°C (350°F).
5. Place the salmon, skin side down, in the air fryer basket. Cook for 6 to 8 minutes, or until the fish flakes in the center.
6. Remove the salmon and plate it on a serving platter. Squeeze fresh lemon over the top of the salmon.
7. Serve immediately.

Basil Crab Cakes With Fresh Salad

Servings: 2

Cooking Time: 25 Minutes

Ingredients:

- 225g lump crabmeat
- 30ml mayonnaise
- ½ tsp Dijon mustard
- ½ tsp lemon juice
- ½ tsp lemon zest
- 2 tsp minced yellow onion
- ¼ tsp prepared horseradish
- 30g flour
- 1 egg white, beaten
- 15g basil, minced
- 15ml olive oil
- 10ml white wine vinegar
- Salt and pepper to taste
- 115g arugula
- 125g blackberries
- 30g pine nuts
- 2 lemon wedges

Directions:

1. Preheat the air fryer to 200°C (400°F).
2. In a bowl, combine the crabmeat, mayonnaise, Dijon mustard, lemon juice, lemon zest, onion, horseradish, flour, beaten egg white, and minced basil to form a mixture.
3. Shape the mixture into 4 patties.
4. Place the patties in the lightly greased air fryer basket.
5. Air Fry for 10 minutes, flipping once during cooking.
6. In another bowl, combine olive oil, white wine vinegar, salt, and pepper. Toss in the arugula and divide it into 2 medium bowls.
7. Add 2 crab cakes to each bowl and scatter with blackberries, pine nuts, and lemon wedges.
8. Serve warm.

Mahi-mahi "burrito" Fillets

Servings: 3

Cooking Time: 10 Minutes

Ingredients:

- 1 large egg white
- 90 grams crushed corn tortilla chips (gluten-free, if needed)
- 5 grams chile powder
- 3 skinless mahi-mahi fillets (approximately 140 grams each)
- 90 grams canned refried beans
- Vegetable oil spray

Directions:

1. Preheat the air fryer to 200°C (400°F).
2. Set up and fill two shallow soup plates or small pie plates on your counter: one with the egg white, beaten until foamy, and one with the crushed tortilla chips.
3. Gently rub 1/2 teaspoon of chile powder on each side of each fillet.
4. Spread 1 tablespoon of refried beans over both sides and the edges of a fillet. Dip the fillet in the egg white, turning to coat it on both sides. Let any excess egg white slip back into the rest, then set the fillet in the crushed tortilla chips. Turn several times, pressing gently to coat it evenly. Coat the fillet on all sides with the vegetable oil spray, then set it aside. Prepare the remaining fillet(s) in the same way.
5. When the air fryer reaches the desired temperature, place the fillets in the basket with as much air space between them as possible. Air-fry undisturbed for 10 minutes, or until they are crisp and browned.
6. Use a nonstick-safe spatula to transfer the fillets to a serving platter or plates. Allow them to cool for only a minute or so, then serve hot.

Basil Mushroom & Shrimp Spaghetti

Servings: 6

Cooking Time: 20 Minutes

Ingredients:

- 225g baby Bella mushrooms, sliced
- 120g grated Parmesan
- 450g peeled shrimp, deveined
- 45ml olive oil
- 1g garlic powder
- 1g shallot powder
- 1g cayenne pepper
- 450g cooked spaghetti pasta
- 5 garlic cloves, minced
- Salt and pepper to taste
- 15g fresh dill

Directions:

1. Preheat the air fryer to 190°C (380°F).
2. Toss the shrimp, 15ml (1 tablespoon) of olive oil, garlic powder, shallot powder, and cayenne pepper in a bowl.
3. Place the seasoned shrimp into the air fryer basket and Roast for 5 minutes. Remove and set aside.
4. In a large skillet over medium heat, warm the remaining olive oil (30ml).
5. Add the minced garlic and sliced mushrooms, and cook for 5 minutes.
6. Pour in the cooked spaghetti pasta, 120ml (½ cup) of water, grated Parmesan, salt, pepper, and fresh dill. Stir to coat the pasta.
7. Stir in the cooked shrimp.
8. Remove from heat and let the mixture rest for 5 minutes.
9. Serve and enjoy your Basil Mushroom & Shrimp Spaghetti!

Malaysian Shrimp With Sambal Mayo

Servings: 4

Cooking Time: 30 Minutes

Ingredients:

- 24 jumbo shrimp, peeled and deveined
- 150 grams panko breadcrumbs
- 3 tablespoons mayonnaise
- 1 tablespoon sambal oelek paste
- 60 grams shredded coconut
- 1 lime, zested
- 1/2 teaspoon ground coriander
- Salt to taste
- 30 grams all-purpose flour
- 2 eggs

Directions:

1. In a bowl, mix together mayonnaise and sambal oelek. Set aside.
2. In another bowl, combine shredded coconut, lime zest, ground coriander, panko breadcrumbs, and salt.
3. In a shallow bowl, place the all-purpose flour. In another shallow bowl, whisk the eggs until well blended.
4. Season the shrimp with salt. Dip each shrimp into the flour, shaking off the excess. Then dip it into the beaten eggs, allowing any excess to drip off. Finally, coat the shrimp with the coconut and panko breadcrumb mixture, pressing gently to adhere.
5. Preheat the air fryer to 180°C (360°F).
6. Place the coated shrimp in the greased frying basket of the air fryer. Cook for 8 minutes, flipping the shrimp once during cooking, until the crust is golden brown and the shrimp is cooked through.
7. Serve the Malaysian shrimp alongside the sambal mayo for dipping.

Dilly Red Snapper

Servings: 4

Cooking Time: 40 Minutes

Ingredients:

- Salt and pepper to taste
- 1/2 tsp ground cumin
- 1/4 tsp cayenne pepper
- 1/4 tsp paprika
- 1 whole red snapper
- 30 grams butter
- 2 garlic cloves, minced
- 15 grams dill
- 4 lemon wedges

Directions:

1. Preheat the air fryer to 180°C (360°F).
2. In a bowl, combine salt, pepper, ground cumin, paprika, and cayenne pepper.
3. Brush the red snapper with butter, then rub it with the seasoning mixture.
4. Stuff the minced garlic and dill inside the cavity of the fish.
5. Place the red snapper into the basket of the air fryer.
6. Roast for 20 minutes, then flip the snapper over and roast for an additional 15 minutes or until the fish is cooked through and has a golden brown exterior.
7. Serve the Dilly Red Snapper with lemon wedges.

Halibut With Coleslaw

Servings: 4

Cooking Time: 30 Minutes

Ingredients:

- 1 bag coleslaw mix
- 60 milliliters mayonnaise
- 5 milliliters lemon zest
- 15 milliliters lemon juice
- 1 shredded carrot
- 120 milliliters buttermilk
- 5 milliliters grated onion
- 4 halibut fillets
- Salt and pepper to taste

Directions:

1. In a bowl, combine the coleslaw mix, mayonnaise, shredded carrot, buttermilk, grated onion, lemon zest, lemon juice, and season with salt to taste. Cover the coleslaw and refrigerate until ready to use.
2. Preheat the air fryer to 180°C (350°F).
3. Sprinkle the halibut fillets with salt and pepper.
4. Grease the air fryer basket, then place the seasoned halibut fillets in it.
5. Air fry for 10 minutes, or until the fillets are opaque and flake easily with a fork.
6. Serve the cooked halibut with the chilled coleslaw.

Bbq Fried Oysters

Servings: 2

Cooking Time: 30 Minutes

Ingredients:

- 60g all-purpose flour
- 120ml barbecue sauce
- 125g bread crumbs
- 225g shelled raw oysters
- 1 lemon
- 15ml chopped parsley

Directions:

1. Preheat the air fryer to 200°C (400°F).
2. In a bowl, place the all-purpose flour.
3. In another bowl, pour the barbecue sauce.
4. In a third bowl, add the breadcrumbs.
5. Roll the shelled raw oysters in the flour, shaking off any excess flour.
6. Dip the floured oysters in the barbecue sauce, shaking off any excess sauce.
7. Dredge the sauced oysters in the breadcrumbs.
8. Place the oysters in the greased air fryer basket.
9. Air Fry for 8 minutes, flipping once during cooking.
10. Sprinkle with chopped parsley and squeeze lemon juice to serve.

Coconut Jerk Shrimp

Servings: 3

Cooking Time: 8 Minutes

Ingredients:

- 1 Large egg white(s)
- 5ml Purchased or homemade jerk dried seasoning blend (see the headnote)
- 90g Plain panko bread crumbs (gluten-free, if a concern)
- 90g Unsweetened shredded coconut
- 12 Large shrimp (20–25 per pound), peeled and deveined
- Coconut oil spray

Directions:

1. Preheat your air fryer to 190°C (375°F).
2. Whisk the egg white(s) and jerk seasoning blend in a bowl until foamy. Add the shrimp and toss well to coat evenly.
3. Mix the bread crumbs and shredded coconut on a dinner plate until well combined. Use kitchen tongs to pick up a shrimp, letting the excess egg white mixture slip back into the bowl. Set the shrimp in the bread-crumb mixture. Turn several times to coat evenly and thoroughly. Set on a cutting board and continue coating the remainder of the shrimp.
4. Lightly coat all the shrimp on both sides with coconut oil spray. Set them in the air fryer basket in one layer with as much space between them as possible. You can even stand some up along the basket's wall in some models.
5. Air-fry undisturbed for 6 minutes, or until the coating is lightly browned. If the air fryer is at 180°C (360°F), you may need to add 2 minutes to the cooking time.
6. Use clean kitchen tongs to transfer the shrimp to a wire rack. Cool for only a minute or two before serving.

Mahi Mahi With Cilantro-chili Butter

Servings: 4

Cooking Time: 20 Minutes

Ingredients:

- Salt and pepper to taste
- 4 mahi-mahi fillets
- 30 grams butter, melted
- 2 garlic cloves, minced
- 1.25 milliliters chili powder
- 1.25 milliliters lemon zest
- 5 grams ginger, minced
- 5 milliliters Worcestershire sauce
- 15 milliliters lemon juice
- 15 grams chopped cilantro

Directions:

1. Preheat the air fryer to 190°C (375°F).
2. Combine melted butter, Worcestershire sauce, minced garlic, salt, lemon juice, minced ginger, black pepper, lemon zest, and chili powder in a small bowl.
3. Place the mahi-mahi fillets on a large plate, then spread the seasoned butter mixture on top of each fillet.
4. Arrange the fish in a single layer in the parchment-lined air fryer basket.
5. Air fry for 6 minutes, then carefully flip the fish. Air fry for another 6-7 minutes until the fish is flaky and cooked through.
6. Serve immediately, sprinkled with chopped cilantro.

Herb-rubbed Salmon With Avocado

Servings: 4

Cooking Time: 30 Minutes

Ingredients:

- 15 milliliters sweet paprika
- 2.5 milliliters cayenne pepper
- 5 milliliters garlic powder
- 5 milliliters dried oregano
- 2.5 milliliters dried coriander
- 5 milliliters dried thyme
- 2.5 milliliters dried dill
- Salt and pepper to taste
- 4 wild salmon fillets
- 30 milliliters chopped red onion
- 22.5 milliliters fresh lemon juice
- 5 milliliters olive oil
- 30 milliliters cilantro, chopped
- 1 avocado, diced

Directions:

1. In a small bowl, mix together the sweet paprika, cayenne pepper, garlic powder, dried oregano, dried thyme, dried dill, dried coriander, salt, and pepper.
2. Spray both sides of the salmon fillets with cooking oil and rub the spice mixture onto the fillets.
3. In a separate bowl, combine the chopped red onion, fresh lemon juice, olive oil, cilantro, salt, and pepper. Allow it to sit for 5 minutes, then gently fold in the diced avocado.
4. Preheat the air fryer to 200°C (400°F).
5. Place the salmon fillets skin-side down in the greased air fryer basket.
6. Air fry for 5-7 minutes or until the fish flakes easily with a fork.
7. Transfer the salmon to a plate and top with the avocado salsa.

Black Cod With Grapes, Fennel, Pecans, And Kale

Servings: 2

Cooking Time: 15 Minutes

Ingredients:

- 2 (170-225g) fillets of black cod (or sablefish)
- Salt and freshly ground black pepper
- Olive oil
- 200g grapes, halved
- 1 small bulb fennel, sliced 6mm thick
- 60g pecans
- 300g shredded kale
- 2 teaspoons white balsamic vinegar or white wine vinegar
- 30ml extra virgin olive oil

Directions:

1. Preheat the air fryer to 200°C (400°F).
2. Season the cod fillets with salt and pepper and drizzle, brush, or spray a little olive oil on top. Place the fish, presentation side up (skin side down), into the air fryer basket. Air-fry for 10 minutes.
3. When the fish has finished cooking, remove the fillets to a side plate and loosely tent with foil to rest.
4. Toss the grapes, fennel, and pecans in a bowl with a drizzle of olive oil and season with salt and pepper. Add the grapes, fennel, and pecans to the air fryer basket and air-fry for 5 minutes at 200°C (400°F), shaking the basket once during the cooking time.
5. Transfer the grapes, fennel, and pecans to a bowl with the kale. Dress the kale with the balsamic vinegar and olive oil, season to taste with salt and pepper, and serve alongside the cooked fish.

Californian Tilapia

Servings: 4

Cooking Time: 15 Minutes

Ingredients:

- Salt and pepper to taste
- 1/4 tsp garlic powder
- 1/4 tsp chili powder
- 1/4 tsp dried oregano
- 1/4 tsp smoked paprika
- 14g butter, melted
- 4 tilapia fillets
- 30ml lime juice
- 1 lemon, sliced

Directions:

1. Preheat your air fryer to 200°C (400°F).
2. In a small bowl, combine salt, pepper, oregano, garlic powder, chili powder, and paprika to create a spice blend.
3. Place the tilapia fillets in a pie pan or similar dish and pour the lime juice and melted butter over the fish.
4. Season both sides of the tilapia fillets with the prepared spice blend.
5. Arrange the seasoned tilapia fillets in a single layer in the parchment-lined air fryer basket, making sure they are not touching each other.
6. Air fry for 4 minutes, then carefully flip the fish.
7. Air fry for an additional 4 to 5 minutes or until the fish is cooked through, and the outside is crispy.
8. Serve your Californian Tilapia immediately with lemon slices on the side.

Lime Flaming Halibut

Servings: 2

Cooking Time: 20 Minutes

Ingredients:

- 30 milliliters butter, melted
- 2.5 milliliters chili powder
- 120 grams bread crumbs
- 2 halibut fillets

Directions:

1. Preheat the air fryer to 180°C (350°F).
2. In a bowl, mix the melted butter, chili powder, and bread crumbs.
3. Press the breadcrumb mixture onto the tops of the halibut fillets.
4. Place the halibut fillets in the greased air fryer basket.
5. Air fry for 10 minutes or until the fish is opaque and flakes easily with a fork.
6. Serve the Lime Flaming Halibut right away.

Hot Calamari Rings

Servings: 4

Cooking Time: 25 Minutes

Ingredients:

- 60 grams all-purpose flour
- 10 milliliters hot chili powder
- 2 eggs
- 15 milliliters milk
- 120 grams bread crumbs
- Salt and pepper to taste
- 450 grams calamari rings
- 1 lime, quartered
- 120 milliliters aioli sauce

Directions:

1. Preheat the air fryer to 200°C (400°F).
2. In a shallow bowl, combine the all-purpose flour and hot chili powder.
3. In another bowl, mix the eggs and milk.
4. In a third bowl, combine the breadcrumbs, salt, and pepper.
5. Dip the calamari rings in the flour mixture first, then in the egg mixture, shaking off any excess, and finally roll them in the breadcrumb mixture.
6. Place the coated calamari rings in the greased air fryer basket.
7. Air fry for 4 minutes, tossing them once during cooking, until they are crispy and golden.
8. Squeeze the lime quarters over the calamari.
9. Serve the hot calamari rings with aioli sauce.

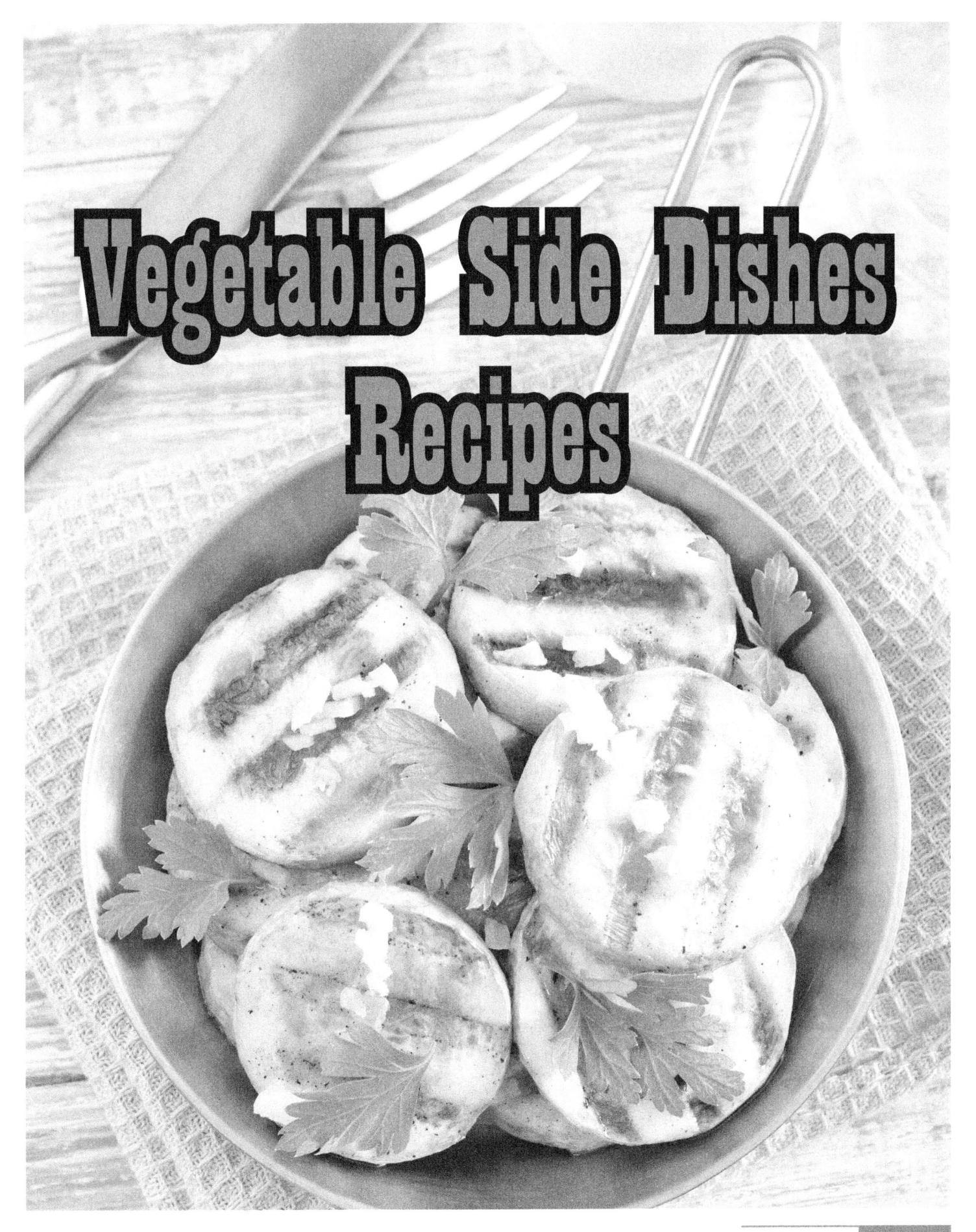

Vegetable Side Dishes Recipes

Vegetable Side Dishes Recipes

Roasted Brussels Sprouts With Bacon

Servings: 4

Cooking Time: 20 Minutes

Ingredients:

- 4 slices of thick-cut bacon, chopped (about 115g)
- 450g Brussels sprouts, halved (or quartered if large)
- Freshly ground black pepper

Directions:

1. Preheat the air fryer to 193°C (380°F).
2. Place the chopped bacon in the air fryer basket. Air-fry the bacon for 5 minutes, shaking the basket once or twice during the cooking time.
3. Add the Brussels sprouts to the basket and drizzle a little bacon fat from the bottom of the air fryer drawer into the basket. Toss the Brussels sprouts to coat them with the bacon fat.
4. Air-fry for an additional 15 minutes or until the Brussels sprouts are tender and can be pierced easily with a knife.
5. Season the roasted Brussels sprouts and bacon with freshly ground black pepper.

Asiago Broccoli

Servings: 4

Cooking Time: 14 Minutes

Ingredients:

- 1 head broccoli, cut into florets
- 15 ml extra-virgin olive oil
- 5 ml minced garlic
- 1 ml ground black pepper
- 1 ml salt
- 30 grams asiago cheese

Directions:

1. Preheat the air fryer to 180°C (360°F).
2. In a medium bowl, toss the broccoli florets with the olive oil, minced garlic, black pepper, and salt.
3. Lightly spray the air fryer basket with olive oil spray.
4. Place the broccoli florets into the basket and cook for 7 minutes.
5. Shake the basket and sprinkle the broccoli with asiago cheese.
6. Cook for an additional 7 minutes.
7. Remove from the basket and serve the Asiago Broccoli warm. Enjoy!

Balsamic Beet Chips

Servings: 4

Cooking Time: 40 Minutes

Ingredients:

- 2.5 ml balsamic vinegar
- 4 beets, peeled and sliced
- 1 garlic clove, minced
- 30 ml chopped mint
- Salt and pepper to taste
- 45 ml olive oil

Directions:

1. Preheat your air fryer to 190°C (380°F).
2. In a bowl, toss all the ingredients together, excluding the balsamic vinegar.
3. Place the beet mixture in the air fryer basket.
4. Roast for 25-30 minutes, stirring once during cooking.
5. Serve the beet chips, drizzled with balsamic vinegar. Enjoy your Balsamic Beet Chips!

Hush Puppies

Servings: 8

Cooking Time: 11 Minutes

Ingredients:

- 120ml Whole or low-fat milk (not fat-free)
- 22.5g Butter
- 120g plus 15g All-purpose flour
- 120g plus 15g Yellow cornmeal
- 10g Granulated white sugar
- 10g Baking powder
- 3.75g Baking soda
- 1.875g Table salt
- 1.25g Onion powder
- 45ml Pasteurized egg substitute (equivalent to 1 medium egg), such as Egg Beaters
- Vegetable oil spray

Directions:

1. Heat the milk and butter in a small saucepan set over medium heat just until the butter melts and the milk is steamy. Do not simmer or boil.
2. Meanwhile, whisk together 120g of flour, 120g of cornmeal, sugar, baking powder, baking soda, salt, and onion powder in a large bowl until the mixture is a uniform color.
3. Stir the hot milk mixture into the flour mixture to form a dough. Set it aside to cool for 5 minutes.
4. Mix the egg substitute or egg into the dough to make a thick, smooth batter. Cover and refrigerate for at least 1 hour or up to 4 hours.
5. Preheat the air fryer to 175°C (350°F).
6. Lightly flour your clean, dry hands. Roll 2 tablespoons of the batter into a ball between your floured palms. Set it aside, flour your hands again if necessary, and continue making more balls with the remaining batter.
7. Coat the balls all over with vegetable oil spray.
8. Line the air fryer basket with a piece of parchment paper. Set the balls on the parchment paper with as much air space between them as possible.
9. Air-fry for 9 minutes, or until lightly browned and set.
10. Use kitchen tongs to gently transfer the hush puppies to a wire rack.
11. Cool for at least 5 minutes before serving. Alternatively, cool to room temperature, about 45 minutes, and store in a sealed container at room temperature for up to 2 days. To crisp the hush puppies again, put them in a 175°C air fryer for 2 minutes. (There's no need for parchment paper in the machine during reheating.)

Mashed Sweet Potato Tots

Servings: 18

Cooking Time: 12 Minutes

Ingredients:

- 240ml cooked mashed sweet potatoes
- 1 egg white, beaten
- 0.625ml ground cinnamon
- A dash of nutmeg
- 30ml chopped pecans
- 7.5ml honey
- Salt
- 120ml panko breadcrumbs
- Oil for misting or cooking spray

Directions:

1. Preheat the air fryer to 200°C (390°F).
2. In a large bowl, mix together the mashed sweet potatoes, beaten egg white, ground cinnamon, nutmeg, chopped pecans, honey, and salt to taste.
3. Place the panko breadcrumbs on a sheet of wax paper.
4. For each tot, use about 2 teaspoons of the sweet potato mixture. To shape, drop the measured potato mixture onto the panko crumbs and push the crumbs up and around the potatoes to coat the edges. Then turn the tot over to coat the other side with crumbs.
5. Mist the tots with oil or cooking spray and place them in the air fryer basket in a single layer.
6. Cook at 200°C (390°F) for 12 minutes, or until they are browned and crispy.
7. Repeat steps 4 and 5 to cook the remaining tots.

Honey-roasted Parsnips

Servings: 3

Cooking Time: 23 Minutes

Ingredients:

- 680g Medium parsnips, peeled
- Olive oil spray
- 15ml Honey
- 7.5ml Water
- 1.25ml Table salt

Directions:

1. Preheat the air fryer to 175°C (350°F).
2. If the thick end of a parsnip is more than 1.25cm (½ inch) in diameter, cut the parsnip just below where it swells to its large end, then slice the large section in half lengthwise. If the parsnips are larger than the basket (or basket attachment), trim off the thin end so the parsnips will fit.
3. Generously coat the parsnips on all sides with olive oil spray.
4. When the air fryer reaches the desired temperature, set the parsnips in the basket with as much air space between them as possible.
5. Air-fry undisturbed for 20 minutes.
6. In a small bowl, whisk together the honey, water, and salt until smooth.
7. Brush this honey mixture over the parsnips.
8. Air-fry undisturbed for 3 minutes more, or until the glaze is lightly browned.
9. Use kitchen tongs to transfer the honey-roasted parsnips to a wire rack or a serving platter.
10. Allow them to cool for a couple of minutes before serving.

Cheese Sage Cauliflower

Servings: 4

Cooking Time: 25 Minutes

Ingredients:

- 1 head cauliflower, cut into florets
- 45 ml butter, melted
- 30 ml grated asiago cheese
- 10 ml dried sage
- 2.5 ml garlic powder
- 1.25 ml salt

Directions:

1. Preheat your air fryer to 180°C (350°F).
2. In a bowl, mix all the ingredients together.
3. Add the cauliflower mixture to the air fryer basket.
4. Air Fry for 6 minutes, shaking the basket once during cooking.
5. Serve your Cheese Sage Cauliflower immediately. Enjoy!

Za'atar Bell Peppers

Servings: 4

Cooking Time: 40 Minutes

Ingredients:

- 1 red bell pepper
- 1 orange bell pepper
- 1 yellow bell pepper
- 2 tsp Za'atar seasoning
- 1 tbsp lemon zest
- ½ tsp salt

Directions:

1. Preheat your air fryer to 188°C (370°F).
2. Pierce each of the bell peppers a few times with a fork to allow steam to escape during cooking.
3. Place the bell peppers in the greased air fryer basket.
4. Air fry for 12-15 minutes, shaking the basket once during cooking, until the peppers become slightly charred.
5. Remove the bell peppers from the air fryer and place them in a small bowl. Cover the bowl and let the peppers sit for 10 minutes; this will help steam them and make it easier to remove the skins.
6. After 10 minutes, peel the skin off the peppers, remove the seeds, and slice them.
7. Sprinkle the sliced peppers with Za'atar seasoning, lemon zest, and salt.
8. Serve your Za'atar Bell Peppers as a flavorful and colourful side dish.

Tuna Platter

Servings: 4

Cooking Time: 9 Minutes

Ingredients:

- 4 new potatoes, boiled in their jackets
- 120 ml vinaigrette dressing, plus 30 ml (2 tablespoons)
- 225g fresh green beans, cut in half-inch pieces and steamed
- 1 tablespoon Herbes de Provence
- 1 tablespoon minced shallots
- 1 ½ tablespoons tarragon vinegar
- 4 tuna steaks, each ¾-inch thick, about 450g in total
- Salt and pepper
- Salad:
- 200g chopped romaine lettuce
- 12 grape tomatoes, halved lengthwise
- 120g pitted olives (black, green, nicoise, or combination)
- 2 boiled eggs, peeled and halved lengthwise

Directions:

1. Quarter the boiled potatoes and toss them with 15ml (1 tablespoon) of salad dressing.
2. Toss the warm green beans with the other 15ml (1 tablespoon) of salad dressing. Set both aside while you prepare the tuna.
3. Mix together the Herbes de Provence, shallots, and tarragon vinegar, and rub this mixture onto all sides of the tuna. Season the fish to taste with salt and pepper.
4. Preheat your air fryer to 200°C (390°F).
5. Cook the tuna at 200°C (390°F) for 7 minutes and check. If needed, cook for an additional 2 minutes longer, until the tuna is barely pink in the center.
6. Spread the chopped romaine lettuce over a large platter.
7. Slice the tuna steaks into 1.3cm (½-inch) pieces and arrange them in the center of the lettuce.
8. Place the remaining ingredients (potatoes, green beans, grape tomatoes, olives, and boiled eggs) around the tuna on the platter.
9. Diners can create their own plates by selecting what they want from the platter. Pass the remainder of the salad dressing at the table.

Buttery Stuffed Tomatoes

Servings: 6

Cooking Time: 15 Minutes

Ingredients:

- 3 225-gram round tomatoes
- 120 ml plus 15 ml Plain panko bread crumbs (gluten-free, if needed)
- 45 grams Finely grated Parmesan cheese
- 45 grams Butter, melted and cooled
- 4 teaspoons Stemmed and chopped fresh parsley leaves
- 5 ml Minced garlic
- 1.25 ml Table salt
- Up to 1.25 ml Red pepper flakes
- Olive oil spray

Directions:

1. Preheat your air fryer to 190°C (375°F).
2. Cut the tomatoes in half horizontally (across their "equators"), being careful not to cut through the stem ends. Gently squeeze each tomato half over a trash can to remove the seeds and most of the juice, making sure to maintain the round shape and avoid crushing the tomatoes.
3. In a bowl, combine the bread crumbs, grated Parmesan cheese, melted butter, chopped parsley, minced garlic, salt, and red pepper flakes. Stir until the bread crumbs are moistened, and the parsley is evenly distributed in the mixture.
4. Fill each tomato half with the breadcrumb mixture, pressing gently to compact the filling. Spray the tops of the stuffed tomatoes with olive oil.
5. Place the tomatoes cut side up in the air fryer basket, and they may touch each other.
6. Air-fry for 15 minutes, or until the filling is lightly browned and crunchy.
7. Use a nonstick-safe spatula and kitchen tongs for balance to gently transfer the stuffed tomatoes to a platter or cutting board.
8. Allow them to cool for a couple of minutes before serving. Enjoy your Buttery Stuffed Tomatoes!

Fried Eggplant Balls

Servings: 4

Cooking Time: 40 Minutes

Ingredients:

- 1 medium eggplant (about 450 grams)
- Olive oil
- Salt and freshly ground black pepper
- 100 grams grated Parmesan cheese
- 200 grams fresh breadcrumbs
- 30 ml chopped fresh parsley
- 30 ml chopped fresh basil
- 1 clove garlic, minced
- 1 egg, lightly beaten
- 50 grams fine dried breadcrumbs

Directions:

1. Preheat your air fryer to 200°C (400°F).
2. Quarter the eggplant by cutting it in half both lengthwise and horizontally. Make a few slashes in the flesh of the eggplant but not through the skin. Brush the cut surface of the eggplant generously with olive oil and transfer to the air fryer basket, cut side up. Air-fry for 10 minutes. Turn the eggplant quarters cut side down and air-fry for another 15 minutes or until the eggplant is soft all the way through. You may need to rotate the pieces in the air fryer so that they cook evenly. Transfer the eggplant to a cutting board to cool.
3. Place the Parmesan cheese, the fresh breadcrumbs, fresh herbs, garlic, and egg in a food processor. Scoop the flesh out of the eggplant, discarding the skin and any pieces that are tough. You should have about 225-300 grams of eggplant. Add the eggplant to the food processor and process everything together until smooth. Season with salt and pepper. Refrigerate the mixture for at least 30 minutes.
4. Place the dried breadcrumbs into a shallow dish or onto a plate. Scoop heaping tablespoons of the eggplant mixture into the dried breadcrumbs. Roll the dollops of eggplant in the breadcrumbs and then shape them into small balls. You should have 16 to 18 eggplant balls at the end. Refrigerate until you are ready to air-fry.
5. Preheat the air fryer to 175°C (350°F).
6. Spray the eggplant balls and the air fryer basket with olive oil. Air-fry the eggplant balls for 15 minutes, rotating them during the cooking process to brown evenly. Enjoy your Fried Eggplant Balls!

Five-spice Roasted Sweet Potatoes

Servings: 4

Cooking Time: 12 Minutes

Ingredients:

- 2.5 ml ground cinnamon
- 1.25 ml ground cumin
- 1.25 ml paprika
- 5 ml chile powder
- 0.6 ml turmeric
- 2.5 ml salt (optional)
- Freshly ground black pepper
- 2 large sweet potatoes, peeled and cut into 2 cm cubes (about 750 ml)
- 15 ml olive oil

Directions:

1. In a large bowl, mix together the ground cinnamon, ground cumin, paprika, chile powder, turmeric, salt (if using), and freshly ground black pepper to taste.
2. Add the sweet potatoes to the bowl and stir well to coat them with the spice mixture.
3. Drizzle the seasoned sweet potatoes with olive oil and stir until they are evenly coated.
4. Place the seasoned sweet potatoes in the air fryer baking pan or an ovenproof dish that fits inside your air fryer basket.
5. Cook for 6 minutes at 200°C (390°F), then stop and stir well.
6. Continue to cook for an additional 6 minutes or until the sweet potatoes are tender and lightly browned. Enjoy your Five-Spice Roasted Sweet Potatoes!

Butternut Medallions With Honey Butter And Sage

Servings: 2

Cooking Time: 15 Minutes

Ingredients:

- 1 butternut squash, peeled
- Olive oil, in a spray bottle
- Salt and freshly ground black pepper
- 30 grams butter, softened
- 30 ml honey
- Pinch of ground cinnamon
- Pinch of ground nutmeg
- Chopped fresh sage

Directions:

1. Preheat your air fryer to 190°C (370°F).
2. Cut the neck of the butternut squash into discs about 1.25 cm thick. (Use the base of the butternut squash for another purpose.)
3. Brush or spray the butternut squash discs with oil and season them with salt and freshly ground black pepper.
4. Place the butternut discs in the air fryer basket in a single layer, with slight overlap if necessary. Air-fry at 190°C for 5 minutes.
5. While the butternut squash is cooking, combine the softened butter, honey, cinnamon, and nutmeg in a small bowl.
6. Brush this honey butter mixture onto the butternut squash discs, flip them over, and brush the other side as well.
7. Continue to air-fry at 190°C for another 5 minutes. Flip the discs once more, brush with more of the honey butter mixture, and air-fry for an additional 5 minutes until the butternut squash is nicely browned around the edges.
8. Remove the butternut squash from the air fryer and repeat with additional batches if necessary.
9. Transfer the cooked butternut squash medallions to a serving platter, sprinkle them with fresh sage, and serve. Enjoy your Butternut Medallions with Honey Butter and Sage!

Greek-inspired Ratatouille

Servings: 6

Cooking Time: 55 Minutes

Ingredients:

- 150g cherry tomatoes
- 1/2 bulb fennel, finely sliced
- 2 russet potatoes, cubed
- 120g tomatoes, cubed
- 1 eggplant, cubed
- 1 zucchini, cubed
- 1 red onion, chopped
- 1 red bell pepper, chopped
- 2 garlic cloves, minced
- 5ml dried mint
- 5ml dried parsley
- 5ml dried oregano
- Salt and pepper to taste
- 1.25ml red pepper flakes
- 80ml olive oil
- 1 can tomato paste
- 60ml vegetable broth

Directions:

1. Preheat the air fryer to 160°C (320°F).
2. In a large bowl, mix together the potatoes, cherry tomatoes, fennel, eggplant, zucchini, onion, red bell pepper, minced garlic, dried mint, dried parsley, dried oregano, salt, black pepper, and red pepper flakes.
3. In a small bowl, whisk together the olive oil, tomato paste, vegetable broth, and 60ml of water.
4. Toss the vegetable mixture with the prepared olive oil and tomato paste mixture to coat them evenly.
5. Pour the coated vegetables into the air frying basket in a single layer.
6. Roast for 20 minutes, then stir well and spread them out again.
7. Roast for an additional 10 minutes, stir again, and then cook for another 10 minutes or until the vegetables are tender and slightly caramelized.
8. Serve your Greek-Inspired Ratatouille and enjoy!

Moroccan Cauliflower

Servings: 6

Cooking Time: 15 Minutes

Ingredients:

- 15ml curry powder
- 10ml smoky paprika
- 2.5ml ground cumin
- 2.5ml salt
- 1 head cauliflower, cut into bite-size pieces
- 60ml red wine vinegar
- 30ml extra-virgin olive oil
- 30ml chopped parsley

Directions:

1. Preheat the air fryer to 190°C (370°F).
2. In a large bowl, mix the curry powder, smoky paprika, ground cumin, and salt.
3. Add the cauliflower to the bowl and stir to coat with the spice mixture.
4. Pour the red wine vinegar over the cauliflower and continue stirring to combine.
5. Place the cauliflower into the air fryer basket and drizzle olive oil over the top.
6. Cook the cauliflower for 5 minutes, toss, and cook for an additional 5 minutes.
7. Raise the temperature to 200°C (400°F) and continue cooking for 4 to 6 minutes, or until the cauliflower is crispy.
8. Sprinkle with chopped parsley and serve.

Speedy Baked Caprese With Avocado

Servings: 4

Cooking Time: 15 Minutes

Ingredients:

- 115g fresh mozzarella
- 8 cherry tomatoes
- 2 teaspoons olive oil
- 2 halved avocados, pitted
- 1/4 teaspoon salt
- 2 tablespoons fresh basil leaves, torn

Directions:

1. Preheat the air fryer to 190°C (375°F).
2. In a bowl, combine the cherry tomatoes and olive oil. Set aside.
3. Place the halved avocados, cut sides up, in the air fryer basket. Scatter the tomatoes around the avocado halves. Bake for 7 minutes.
4. Divide the baked avocado halves between 4 small plates. Top each avocado half with 2 baked tomatoes and sprinkle with salt.
5. Cut the fresh mozzarella cheese into pieces and evenly distribute them over the baked tomatoes.
6. Scatter torn basil leaves over the top of each plate to serve.

Street Corn

Servings: 4

Cooking Time: 10 Minutes

Ingredients:

- 15g butter
- 4 ears corn
- 80ml plain Greek yogurt
- 30g Parmesan cheese
- 2.5ml paprika
- 2.5ml garlic powder
- 1.25ml salt
- 1.25ml black pepper
- 15g finely chopped cilantro (coriander)

Directions:

1. Preheat your air fryer to 200°C (400°F).
2. In a medium microwave-safe bowl, melt the butter in the microwave. Lightly brush the outside of the ears of corn with the melted butter.
3. Place the corn into the air fryer basket and cook for 5 minutes, flip the corn, and cook for another 5 minutes.
4. Meanwhile, in a medium bowl, mix the yogurt, cheese, paprika, garlic powder, salt, and pepper. Set aside.
5. Carefully remove the corn from the air fryer and let them cool for 3 minutes.
6. Brush the outside edges of the corn with the yogurt mixture and top with fresh chopped cilantro.
7. Serve immediately.

Air Fryer Cookbook

Gorgonzola Stuffed Mushrooms

Servings: 2

Cooking Time: 15 Minutes

Ingredients:

- 12 white button mushroom caps
- 30ml diced white button mushroom stems
- 60ml Gorgonzola cheese, crumbled
- 5ml olive oil
- 1 green onion, chopped
- 30ml bread crumbs

Directions:

1. Preheat the air fryer to 180°C (350°F).
2. Rub a little olive oil around the top of each mushroom cap.
3. In a bowl, mix together the diced mushroom stems, chopped green onion, and crumbled Gorgonzola cheese.
4. Distribute and press the mixture into the cups of the mushroom caps, then sprinkle bread crumbs on top.
5. Place the stuffed mushrooms in the air fryer basket.
6. Air fry for 5-7 minutes until the mushrooms are tender and the cheese is melted.
7. Serve the Gorgonzola Stuffed Mushrooms right away.

Caraway Seed Pretzel Sticks

Servings: 4

Cooking Time: 30 Minutes

Ingredients:

- 225 grams pizza dough
- 5 ml baking soda
- 30 ml caraway seeds

Directions:

1. Preheat your air fryer to 200°C (400°F).
2. Roll out the pizza dough on parchment paper into a rectangle, then cut it into 8 strips.
3. In a bowl, whisk together the baking soda and 240 ml (1 cup) of hot water until well dissolved.
4. Submerge each dough strip into the baking soda solution, shake off any excess, and stretch them another 2.5 to 5 cm (1 to 2 inches).
5. Sprinkle the stretched dough strips with caraway seeds and let them rise for 10 minutes in the air fryer basket.
6. Grease the pretzel sticks with cooking spray.
7. Air Fry for 8 minutes, turning them once during cooking, or until they are golden brown.
8. Serve your Caraway Seed Pretzel Sticks. Enjoy!

Almond-crusted Zucchini Fries

Servings: 2

Cooking Time: 30 Minutes

Ingredients:

- 30 grams grated Pecorino cheese
- 1 zucchini, cut into fries
- 1 teaspoon salt
- 1 egg
- 15 ml almond milk
- 60 grams almond flour

Directions:

1. Preheat the air fryer to 190°C (370°F).
2. Lay out the zucchini fries on a paper towel, sprinkle with salt, and allow them to sit for 10 minutes to draw out moisture. Pat them dry with additional paper towels.
3. In a bowl, beat the egg and almond milk.
4. In another bowl, combine almond flour and grated Pecorino cheese.
5. Dip the zucchini fries into the egg mixture and then coat them with the flour and cheese mixture.
6. Place the coated zucchini fries in the lightly greased frying basket of the air fryer.
7. Air Fry for 10 minutes, flipping the fries once during cooking for even browning.
8. Serve the almond-crusted zucchini fries hot. Enjoy!

Baked Shishito Peppers

Servings: 2

Cooking Time: 15 Minutes

Ingredients:

- 170 grams shishito peppers
- 5 ml olive oil
- 5 ml salt
- 60 ml soy sauce

Directions:

1. Preheat your air fryer to 190°C (375°F).
2. In a mixing bowl, combine all the ingredients.
3. Place the shishito peppers in the air fryer basket.
4. Bake for 8 minutes, or until the peppers are blistered, shaking the basket once during cooking.
5. Serve the baked shishito peppers with soy sauce for dipping. Enjoy!

Fried Eggplant Slices

Servings: 3

Cooking Time: 12 Minutes

Ingredients:

- 1.5 sleeves (about 60 saltines) Saltine crackers
- 175 grams Cornstarch
- 2 Large egg(s), well beaten
- 1 medium (about 340 grams) Eggplant, stemmed, peeled, and cut into 0.6 cm-thick rounds
- Olive oil spray

Directions:

1. Preheat your air fryer to 200°C (400°F). Also, position the rack in the center of the oven and heat the oven to 80°C (175°F).
2. Grind the saltines, in batches if necessary, in a food processor, pulsing the machine and rearranging the saltine pieces every few pulses. Or pulverize the saltines in a large, heavy zip-closed plastic bag with the bottom of a heavy saucepan. In either case, you want small bits of saltines, not just crumbs.
3. Set up and fill three shallow soup plates or small pie plates on your counter: one for the cornstarch, one for the beaten egg(s), and one for the pulverized saltines.
4. Set an eggplant slice in the cornstarch and turn it to coat on both sides. Use a brush to lightly remove any excess. Dip it into the beaten egg(s) and turn to coat both sides. Let any excess egg slip back into the rest, then set the slice in the saltines. Turn several times, pressing gently to coat both sides evenly but not heavily. Coat both sides of the slice with olive oil spray and set it aside. Continue dipping and coating the remaining slices.
5. Set one, two, or maybe three slices in the basket. There should be at least 1.25 cm (½ inch) between them for proper air flow. Air-fry undisturbed for 12 minutes, or until they are crisp and browned.
6. Use a nonstick-safe spatula to transfer the slice(s) to a large baking sheet. Slip them into the oven to keep the slices warm as you air-fry more batches, as needed, always transferring the slices to the baking sheet to stay warm. Enjoy your Fried Eggplant Slices!

Corn On The Cob

Servings: 4

Cooking Time: 12 Minutes

Ingredients:

- 2 large ears fresh corn
- Olive oil for misting
- Salt (optional)

Directions:

1. Shuck the corn, remove the silks, and wash.
2. Cut or break each ear in half crosswise.
3. Spray the corn with olive oil.
4. Cook at 200°C (390°F) for 12 minutes or until browned to your liking.
5. Serve plain or with coarsely ground salt if desired. Enjoy your Corn on the Cob!

Stuffed Onions

Servings: 6

Cooking Time: 27 Minutes

Ingredients:

- 6 Small 100-115g yellow or white onions
- Olive oil spray
- 170g Bulk sweet Italian sausage meat (gluten-free, if needed)
- 9 Cherry tomatoes, chopped
- 3 tablespoons Seasoned Italian-style dried breadcrumbs (gluten-free, if needed)
- 3 tablespoons (about 14g) Finely grated Parmesan cheese

Directions:

1. Preheat the air fryer to 160°C (or 165°C if that's the closest setting).
2. Cut just enough off the root ends of the onions so they will stand up on a cutting board when this end is turned down. Carefully peel off just the brown, papery skin. Now cut the top quarter off each and place the onion back on the cutting board with this end facing up. Use a flatware spoon (preferably a serrated grapefruit spoon) or a melon baller to scoop out the "insides" (interior layers) of the onion, leaving enough of the bottom and side walls so that the onion does not collapse. Depending on the thickness of the layers in the onion, this may be one or two of those layers—or even three if they're very thin.
3. Coat the insides and outsides of the onions with olive oil spray. Set the onion "shells" in the air fryer basket and air-fry for 15 minutes.
4. Meanwhile, make the filling. Set a medium skillet over medium heat for a couple of minutes, then crumble in the sausage meat. Cook, stirring often, until browned, about 4 minutes. Transfer the contents of the skillet to a medium bowl (leave the fat behind in the skillet or add it to the bowl, depending on your preference). Stir in the tomatoes, breadcrumbs, and cheese until well combined.
5. When the onions are ready, use a nonstick-safe spatula to gently transfer them to a cutting board. Increase the air fryer's temperature to 175°C.
6. Pack the sausage mixture into the onion shells, gently compacting the filling and mounding it up at the top.
7. When the machine is at temperature, set the onions stuffing side up in the basket with at least ¼ inch between them. Air-fry for 12 minutes, or until lightly browned and sizzling hot.
8. Use a nonstick-safe spatula, and perhaps a flatware fork for balance, to transfer the onions to a cutting board or serving platter. Cool for 5 minutes before serving.

Turkish Mutabal (eggplant Dip)

Servings: 2

Cooking Time: 40 Minutes

Ingredients:

- 1 medium eggplant
- 2 tablespoons tahini
- 2 tablespoons lemon juice
- 1 teaspoon garlic powder
- ¼ teaspoon sumac
- 1 teaspoon chopped parsley

Directions:

1. Preheat your air fryer to 200°C (400°F).
2. Place the eggplant in a pan and roast it in the air fryer for 30 minutes, turning it once during cooking.
3. Let the roasted eggplant cool for 5-10 minutes.
4. Scoop out the flesh from the eggplant and place it in a bowl.
5. Squeeze out any excess water from the eggplant and discard the water.
6. Mix the eggplant flesh, tahini, lemon juice, garlic powder, and sumac until well combined.
7. Scatter chopped parsley over the dip.
8. Serve your Turkish Mutabal (Eggplant Dip).

Beef, pork & Lamb Recipes

Beef, pork & Lamb Recipes

Blackberry Bbq Glazed Country-style Ribs

Servings: 2

Cooking Time: 40 Minutes

Ingredients:

- 120 ml + 30 ml (1/2 cup + 2 tablespoons) sherry or Madeira wine, divided
- 450 grams (1 pound) boneless country-style pork ribs
- Salt and freshly ground black pepper
- 15 ml (1 tablespoon) Chinese 5-spice powder
- 60 ml (1/4 cup) blackberry preserves
- 60 ml (1/4 cup) hoisin sauce*
- 1 clove garlic, minced
- 1 generous tablespoon grated fresh ginger
- 2 scallions, chopped
- 15 ml (1 tablespoon) sesame seeds, toasted

Directions:

1. Preheat the air fryer to 165°C (330°F) and pour 120 ml (1/2 cup) of the sherry into the bottom of the air fryer drawer.
2. Season the ribs with salt, pepper, and the Chinese 5-spice powder.
3. Air-fry the ribs at 165°C (330°F) for 20 minutes, turning them over halfway through the cooking time.
4. While the ribs are cooking, make the sauce. Combine the remaining 30 ml (2 tablespoons) of sherry, blackberry preserves, hoisin sauce, minced garlic, and grated ginger in a small saucepan. Bring to a simmer on the stovetop for a few minutes until the sauce thickens.
5. When the time is up on the air fryer, turn the ribs over, pour a little sauce on the ribs, and air-fry for another 10 minutes at 165°C (330°F). Turn the ribs over again, pour on more of the sauce, and air-fry at 165°C (330°F) for a final 10 minutes.
6. Let the ribs rest for at least 5 minutes before serving them warm with a little more glaze brushed on and the chopped scallions and toasted sesame seeds sprinkled on top.

Citrus Pork Lettuce Wraps

Servings: 4

Cooking Time: 35 Minutes

Ingredients:

- Salt and white pepper to taste
- 15 ml cornflour
- 15 ml red wine vinegar
- 30 ml orange marmalade
- 5 ml pulp-free orange juice
- 10 ml olive oil
- 1.25 ml chili pepper
- 1.25 ml ground ginger
- 450 g pork loin, cubed
- 8 iceberg lettuce leaves
- Instructions:
- In a bowl, create a slurry by whisking together the cornflour and 15 ml of water. Set it aside.
- Place a small saucepan over medium heat. Add the red wine vinegar, orange marmalade, orange juice, olive oil, chili pepper, and ground ginger. Cook for 3 minutes, stirring continuously.
- Mix in the cornflour slurry and simmer for 1 more minute. Turn off the heat and let it thicken, which should take about 3 minutes.
- Preheat your air fryer to 180°C (350°F).
- Sprinkle the pork with salt and white pepper. Place the pork cubes in the greased frying basket and air fry for 8-10 minutes until they are cooked through and browned, turning them once.
- Transfer the pork cubes to a bowl, add the sauce, and toss to coat.
- To serve, place the sauced pork in the iceberg lettuce leaves, creating wraps. Enjoy your Citrus Pork Lettuce Wraps!

Glazed Meatloaf

Servings: 4

Cooking Time: 35-55 Minutes

Ingredients:

- 65g Seasoned Italian-style panko bread crumbs (gluten-free, if a concern)
- 60ml Whole or low-fat milk
- 450g Lean ground beef
- 450g Bulk mild Italian sausage meat (gluten-free, if a concern)
- 1 Large egg(s), well beaten
- 1 teaspoon Dried thyme
- 1 teaspoon Onion powder
- 1 teaspoon Garlic powder
- Vegetable oil spray
- 15ml Ketchup (gluten-free, if a concern)
- 15ml Hoisin sauce (gluten-free, if a concern)
- 10ml Pickle brine, preferably from a jar of jalapeño rings (gluten-free, if a concern)

Directions:

1. Pour the bread crumbs into a large bowl, add the milk, stir gently, and soak for 10 minutes.
2. Preheat the air fryer to 175°C (350°F).
3. Add the ground beef, Italian sausage meat, egg(s), thyme, onion powder, and garlic powder to the bowl with the bread crumbs. Blend gently until well combined. (Clean, dry hands work best!) Form this mixture into an oval loaf about 5cm tall (its length will vary depending on the amount of ingredients) but with a flat bottom. Generously coat the top, bottom, and all sides of the loaf with vegetable oil spray.
4. Use a large, nonstick-safe spatula or perhaps silicone baking mitts to transfer the loaf to the basket. Air-fry undisturbed for 30 minutes for a small meatloaf, 40 minutes for a medium one, or 50 minutes for a large, until an instant-read meat thermometer inserted into the center of the loaf registers 74°C (165°F).
5. Whisk the ketchup, hoisin, and pickle brine in a small bowl until smooth. Brush this over the top and sides of the meatloaf and continue air-frying undisturbed for 5 minutes, or until the glaze has browned a bit.
6. Use that same spatula or those same baking mitts to transfer the meatloaf to a cutting board. Cool for 10 minutes before slicing.

Balsamic London Broil

Servings: 4

Cooking Time: 25 Minutes

Ingredients:

- 1.13 kilograms top round London broil steak
- 60 ml coconut aminos
- 15 ml balsamic vinegar
- 15 ml olive oil
- 15 ml mustard
- 10 ml maple syrup
- 2 garlic cloves, minced
- 5 grams dried oregano
- Salt and pepper to taste
- 0.6 grams smoked paprika
- 30 grams red onions, chopped

Directions:

1. Whisk together the coconut aminos, mustard, balsamic vinegar, olive oil, maple syrup, minced garlic, dried oregano, chopped red onions, salt, pepper, and smoked paprika in a small bowl to make the marinade.
2. Place the London broil steak in a shallow container and pour the marinade over the steak. Make sure the steak is well coated with the marinade. Cover the container and let it sit for 20 minutes to marinate.
3. Preheat the air fryer to 200°C (400°F).
4. Transfer the marinated steak to the air fryer basket.
5. Air fry for 5 minutes, then flip the steak and air fry for another 4 to 6 minutes, or until the desired level of doneness is reached. Cooking times may vary depending on your air fryer and the thickness of the steak.
6. Allow the cooked steak to rest for 5 minutes before slicing.
7. Serve your Balsamic London Broil warm and enjoy!

Crispy Pork Escalopes

Servings: 4

Cooking Time: 20 Minutes

Ingredients:

- 4 pork loin steaks
- Salt and pepper to taste
- 30g flour
- 2 tbsp bread crumbs

Directions:

1. Preheat the air fryer to 190°C (380°F).
2. Season the pork loin steaks with salt and pepper to taste.
3. In one shallow bowl, add the flour. In another shallow bowl, add the bread crumbs.
4. Dip each pork steak first in the flour, ensuring it's coated evenly, and then in the bread crumbs, pressing lightly to adhere the crumbs to the pork.
5. Place the breaded pork steaks in the preheated air fryer basket in a single layer. Spray them with a light coat of cooking oil.
6. Air fry for 12-14 minutes, flipping the steaks once during cooking, until they are crisp and cooked through.
7. Serve your crispy pork escalopes immediately.

Berbere Beef Steaks

Servings: 4

Cooking Time: 45 Minutes

Ingredients:

- 1 chipotle pepper in adobo sauce, minced
- 450 grams (1 lb) skirt steak
- 30 ml (2 tablespoons) chipotle sauce
- 1/4 teaspoon Berbere seasoning
- Salt and pepper to taste

Directions:

1. Cut the skirt steak into 4 equal pieces and place them on a plate.
2. In a bowl, mix together the minced chipotle pepper, adobo sauce, salt, pepper, and Berbere seasoning.
3. Spread the chipotle mixture on both sides of the steak pieces. Chill the steak in the refrigerator for 2 hours.
4. Preheat the air fryer to 200°C (390°F).
5. Place the marinated steaks in the frying basket of the air fryer and bake for 5 minutes on each side for well-done meat.
6. Allow the steaks to rest for an additional 5 minutes.
7. To serve, slice the steaks against the grain.

Boneless Ribeye Steaks

Servings: 2

Cooking Time: 10-15 Minutes

Ingredients:

- 2 boneless ribeye steaks, approximately 227 grams (8 ounces) each
- 4 teaspoons Worcestershire sauce
- 1/2 teaspoon garlic powder
- Coarsely ground black pepper to taste
- 4 teaspoons extra virgin olive oil
- Salt to taste

Directions:

1. Season both sides of the ribeye steaks with Worcestershire sauce. Use the back of a spoon to spread it evenly.
2. Sprinkle both sides of the steaks with garlic powder and coarsely ground black pepper to taste.
3. Drizzle both sides of the steaks with olive oil, again using the back of a spoon to spread it evenly over the surfaces.
4. Allow the steaks to marinate for 30 minutes.
5. Place both steaks in the air fryer basket and cook at 200°C (390°F) for 5 minutes.
6. Turn the steaks over and cook until done:
7. Medium Rare: Additional 5 minutes
8. Medium: Additional 7 minutes
9. Well Done: Additional 10 minutes
10. Remove the steaks from the air fryer basket and let them sit for 5 minutes. Salt to taste and serve.

Cinnamon-stick Kofta Skewers

Servings: 8

Cooking Time: 15 Minutes

Ingredients:

- 450g Lean ground beef
- 1.25ml Ground cumin
- 1.25ml Onion powder
- 1.25ml Ground dried turmeric
- 1.25ml Ground cinnamon
- 1.25ml Table salt
- Up to 0.3ml Cayenne
- 8 cinnamon sticks, each 9-10cm long
- Vegetable oil spray

Directions:

1. Preheat your air fryer to 190°C (375°F).
2. Gently mix the lean ground beef, ground cumin, onion powder, ground turmeric, ground cinnamon, table salt, and cayenne in a bowl until the meat is evenly mixed with the spices. Use clean, dry hands for mixing.
3. Divide this mixture into 2-ounce portions, each about the size of a golf ball.
4. Wrap one portion of the meat mixture around a cinnamon stick, using about three-quarters of the length of the stick. Cover one end but leave a little "handle" of cinnamon stick protruding from the other end. Set it aside and continue making more kofta skewers.
5. Generously coat the formed kofta skewers on all sides with vegetable oil spray.
6. Set the skewers in the air fryer basket with as much air space between them as possible.
7. Air-fry undisturbed for 13 minutes, or until they are browned and cooked through. If the machine is at 180°C (360°F), you may need to add 2 minutes to the cooking time.
8. Use a nonstick-safe spatula and kitchen tongs if needed to gently transfer the kofta skewers to a wire rack. Allow them to cool for at least 5 minutes or up to 20 minutes before serving.

Asian-style Flank Steak

Servings: 4

Cooking Time: 25 Minutes

Ingredients:

- 450 grams flank steak, cut into strips
- 4 tbsp cornstarch
- Black pepper to taste
- 1 tbsp grated ginger
- 3 garlic cloves, minced
- 150 ml beef stock
- 2 tbsp soy sauce
- 2 tbsp light brown sugar
- 2 scallions, chopped
- 1 tbsp sesame seeds

Directions:

1. Preheat the air fryer to 200°C (400°F).
2. Sprinkle the beef strips with 3 tablespoons of cornstarch and season with black pepper. Toss to coat the beef evenly.
3. Line the frying basket with round parchment paper with holes poked in it to prevent sticking. Place the coated steak in the basket and spray it lightly with cooking oil.
4. Air fry for 8-12 minutes, shaking the basket after 5 minutes to ensure even cooking, until the beef is browned. Remove the beef from the air fryer and set it aside.
5. In a bowl, combine the remaining 1 tablespoon of cornstarch, grated ginger, minced garlic, beef stock, soy sauce, light brown sugar, and chopped scallions.
6. Place the mixture in the frying basket of the air fryer.
7. Air fry for an additional 5-8 minutes, stirring the sauce after 3 minutes, until the sauce is thick and glossy.
8. Plate the cooked beef, pour the sauce over it, toss to coat, and sprinkle with sesame seeds.
9. Serve your Asian-Style Flank Steak and enjoy!

Balsamic Marinated Rib Eye Steak With Balsamic Fried Cipollini Onions

Servings: 2

Cooking Time: 22-26 Minutes

Ingredients:

- 45 ml balsamic vinegar
- 2 cloves garlic, sliced
- 15 ml Dijon mustard
- 5 grams fresh thyme leaves
- 454 grams boneless rib eye steak
- Coarsely ground black pepper
- Salt
- 227 grams cipollini onions, peeled
- 5 ml balsamic vinegar

Directions:

1. In a small bowl, combine 45 ml of balsamic vinegar, sliced garlic, Dijon mustard, and fresh thyme leaves to make the marinade.
2. Pour the marinade over the rib eye steak.
3. Pierce the steak several times with a paring knife or a needle-style meat tenderizer. Season the steak generously with coarsely ground black pepper.
4. Flip the steak over and pierce the other side in a similar fashion, seasoning again with coarsely ground black pepper.
5. Marinate the steak for 2 to 24 hours in the refrigerator.
6. When you're ready to cook, remove the steak from the refrigerator and let it sit at room temperature for 30 minutes.
7. Preheat the air fryer to 200°C (400°F).
8. Season the steak with salt and air-fry at 200°C (400°F) for 12 minutes (medium-rare), 14 minutes (medium), or 16 minutes (well-done), flipping the steak once halfway through the cooking time.
9. While the steak is air-frying, toss the peeled cipollini onions with 5 ml of balsamic vinegar and season with salt.
10. Remove the steak from the air fryer and let it rest while you fry the onions.
11. Transfer the seasoned onions to the air fryer basket and air-fry for 10 minutes, adding a few more minutes if your onions are very large.
12. Afterward, slice the steak on the bias and serve with the fried onions on top.

Egg Stuffed Pork Meatballs

Servings: 2

Cooking Time: 40 Minutes

Ingredients:

- 3 soft-boiled eggs, peeled
- 225g ground pork
- 2 tsp dried tarragon
- ½ tsp hot paprika
- 2 tsp garlic powder
- Salt and pepper to taste

Directions:

1. Preheat your air fryer to 175°C (350°F).
2. In a mixing bowl, combine the ground pork, dried tarragon, hot paprika, garlic powder, and season with salt and pepper to taste. Mix well until all the spices are evenly distributed throughout the meat.
3. Divide the pork mixture into three equal portions in the mixing bowl.
4. Take one portion of the pork mixture and flatten it on a clean work surface to create a wide, flat meat circle.
5. Place one soft-boiled egg in the center of the meat circle.
6. Use your hands to carefully mold the pork mixture up and around the egg, ensuring it's completely enclosed by the meat. Repeat this process for the remaining two eggs.
7. Place the stuffed meatballs in the air fryer basket, ensuring they have some space between them for even cooking.
8. Air fry the meatballs at 175°C (350°F) for 18-20 minutes, shaking the basket once during cooking to ensure even browning and crispiness.
9. Once the meatballs are crispy and golden brown, remove them from the air fryer.
10. Allow the Egg Stuffed Pork Meatballs to cool slightly, and then serve.

Carne Asada Recipes

Servings: 4

Cooking Time: 15 Minutes

Ingredients:

- 4 cloves garlic, minced
- 3 chipotle peppers in adobo, chopped
- 80ml chopped fresh parsley
- 80ml chopped fresh oregano
- 5ml ground cumin seed
- Juice of 2 limes
- 80ml olive oil
- 450g to 680g flank steak (depending on your appetite)
- Salt
- Tortillas and guacamole (optional – for serving)

Directions:

1. Make the marinade: Combine the minced garlic, chopped chipotle peppers, fresh parsley, fresh oregano, ground cumin, lime juice, and olive oil in a non-reactive bowl.
2. Coat the flank steak with the marinade and let it marinate for 30 minutes to 8 hours. Make sure not to leave the steak out of refrigeration for longer than 2 hours.
3. Preheat your air fryer to 200°C (390°F).
4. Remove the steak from the marinade and place it in the air fryer basket.
5. Season the steak with salt.
6. Air-fry the steak for 15 minutes, turning the steak over halfway through the cooking time and seasoning it again with salt. This should cook the steak to medium. Adjust the time by adding or subtracting two minutes for medium-well or medium-rare, depending on your preference.
7. Remember to let the steak rest before slicing the meat against the grain.
8. Serve your Carne Asada with warm tortillas, guacamole, and a fresh salsa, like the Tomato-Corn Salsa below.

Beef Brazilian Empanadas

Servings: 6

Cooking Time: 40 Minutes

Ingredients:

- 120g shredded Pepper Jack cheese
- 1/3 minced green bell pepper
- 120g shredded mozzarella
- 2 garlic cloves, chopped
- 1/3 onion, chopped
- 225g ground beef
- 1 teaspoon allspice
- ½ teaspoon paprika
- ½ teaspoon chili powder
- Salt and pepper to taste
- 15 empanada wrappers
- 15ml butter

Directions:

1. Spray a skillet with cooking oil. Over medium heat, stir-fry the chopped garlic, minced green bell pepper, and chopped onion for 2 minutes or until aromatic.
2. Add the ground beef, allspice, chili powder, paprika, salt, and pepper. Use a spoon to break up the beef. Cook until it's browned. Drain the excess fat.
3. On a clean work surface, glaze the edge of each empanada wrapper with water using a basting brush to soften the crust.
4. Mound 2-3 tablespoons of the cooked beef mixture onto each wrapper.
5. Top the beef with mozzarella and Pepper Jack cheese.
6. Fold one side of the wrapper over to the opposite side, creating a half-moon shape. Press the edges with the back of a fork to seal the empanadas.
7. Preheat the air fryer to 200°C (400°F).
8. Place the empanadas in the air fryer and spray them with cooking oil.
9. Bake for 8 minutes, then flip the empanadas.
10. Cook for another 4 minutes until they are golden and crispy.
11. Melt the butter in a microwave-safe bowl for 20 seconds. Brush the melted butter over the top of each empanada.
12. Serve your Beef Brazilian Empanadas warm and enjoy!

Homemade Pork Gyoza

Servings: 4

Cooking Time: 50 Minutes

Ingredients:

- 8 wonton wrappers
- 115g ground pork, browned
- 1 green apple
- 5ml rice vinegar
- 15ml vegetable oil
- 7.5ml oyster sauce
- 15ml soy sauce
- A pinch of white pepper

Directions:

1. Preheat your air fryer to 180°C (350°F).
2. In a small bowl, combine the oyster sauce, soy sauce, rice vinegar, and a pinch of white pepper. Add the browned ground pork and mix thoroughly.
3. Peel and core the green apple, then slice it into small cubes. Add the apple cubes to the pork mixture and combine well.
4. Lay out the wonton wrappers and place a portion of the pork and apple filling in the center of each wrapper.
5. Moisten the edges of the wrappers with a bit of water and fold them into triangles, pressing the edges to seal.
6. Brush the sealed gyoza with vegetable oil to help them crisp up.
7. Place the gyoza in the air fryer basket in a single layer, making sure they do not touch each other.
8. Air fry for about 25 minutes until the gyoza turn crispy golden brown on the outside and are cooked through.
9. Serve your homemade pork gyoza hot with your favorite dipping sauce, and enjoy the delicious flavors!

Carne Asada

Servings: 3

Cooking Time: 12 Minutes

Ingredients:

- 60ml Orange juice
- 3 tablespoons Regular or low-sodium soy sauce or gluten-free tamari sauce
- 22.5ml Lemon juice
- 22.5ml Lime juice
- 7.5ml Minced garlic
- 3.75ml Ground cumin
- 3.75ml Dried oregano
- Up to 3.75ml Red pepper flakes
- 340g Beef skirt steak

Directions:

1. In a large bowl, mix together the orange juice, soy sauce or tamari sauce, lemon juice, lime juice, minced garlic, ground cumin, dried oregano, and red pepper flakes.
2. Add the skirt steak to the marinade, turning it several times to coat. Cover and refrigerate for at least 2 hours, up to 6 hours, turning the meat in the marinade two or more times.
3. Preheat your air fryer to 200°C (400°F).
4. Meanwhile, remove the steak from the marinade, discard any remaining marinade, and cut the steak into pieces that will fit in the basket in a single layer. Leave these pieces out at room temperature as the machine heats.
5. Once the air fryer reaches the desired temperature, set the steak pieces in the basket, overlapping them as necessary without letting any climb up the side of the basket.
6. Air-fry for 12 minutes, turning and rearranging the pieces once to ensure even cooking, until they are browned and sizzling.
7. Use kitchen tongs to transfer the pieces of skirt steak to a cutting board. Let them cool for 5 minutes, then carve them against the grain into 1.25cm (½ inch) thick strips.

Cajun Pork Loin Chops

Servings: 4

Cooking Time: 25 Minutes

Ingredients:

- 8 thin boneless pork loin chops
- ¾ teaspoon Coarse sea salt
- 1 egg, beaten
- 1 teaspoon Cajun seasoning
- 60g bread crumbs
- 1 cucumber, sliced
- 1 tomato, sliced

Directions:

1. Place the pork chops between two sheets of parchment paper. Pound the pork to a thickness of approximately 6mm (¼ inch) using a meat mallet or rolling pin. Season the pork chops with sea salt.
2. In a shallow bowl, beat the egg with 5ml (1 teaspoon) of water and the Cajun seasoning.
3. In a second bowl, place the breadcrumbs.
4. Dip each pork chop into the egg mixture, allowing any excess to drip off, and then dip it into the breadcrumbs to coat it evenly.
5. Preheat your air fryer to 200°C (400°F).
6. Grease the air fryer frying basket and place the coated pork chops in it.
7. Air fry for 6-8 minutes, flipping the chops once during cooking, until they are golden and cooked through.
8. Serve the Cajun Pork Loin Chops immediately, accompanied by sliced cucumber and tomato.

Chipotle Pork Meatballs

Servings: 4

Cooking Time: 35 Minutes

Ingredients:

- 450g ground pork
- 1 egg
- 60ml chipotle sauce
- 60ml grated celery
- 60ml chopped parsley
- 60ml chopped cilantro
- 60ml flour
- 1.25ml salt

Directions:

1. Preheat your air fryer to 180°C (350°F).
2. In a large bowl, combine the ground pork, egg, chipotle sauce, grated celery, chopped parsley, chopped cilantro, flour, and salt.
3. Form the mixture into 16 meatballs.
4. Place the meatballs in the lightly greased frying basket of the air fryer.
5. Air fry for 8-10 minutes, flipping the meatballs once to ensure even cooking.
6. Serve the Chipotle Pork Meatballs immediately!

Garlic-buttered Rib Eye Steak

Servings: 2

Cooking Time: 25 Minutes

Ingredients:

- 450g rib eye steak
- Salt and pepper to taste
- 15g butter
- 5g paprika
- 15g chopped rosemary
- 2 garlic cloves, minced
- 30g chopped parsley
- 15g chopped mint

Directions:

1. Preheat your air fryer to 200°C (400°F).
2. Season both sides of the rib eye steak with salt and pepper.
3. Place the seasoned rib eye steak in the greased air fryer basket.
4. Top the steak with butter, minced garlic, paprika, chopped rosemary, and chopped mint.
5. Air fry for 6 minutes, then flip the steak and air fry for an additional 6 minutes. For a medium-rare steak, the internal temperature should reach 60°C (140°F).
6. Remove the steak from the air fryer and let it rest for 5 minutes.
7. Sprinkle the cooked steak with chopped parsley.
8. Slice the steak and serve immediately. Enjoy your Garlic-Buttered Rib Eye Steak!

French-style Steak Salad

Servings: 4

Cooking Time: 25 Minutes

Ingredients:

- 250g sliced strawberries
- 60g crumbled blue cheese
- 60ml olive oil
- Salt and pepper to taste
- 1 flank steak
- 60ml balsamic vinaigrette
- 15ml Dijon mustard
- 30ml lemon juice
- 200g baby arugula
- 1/2 red onion, sliced
- 60g pecan pieces
- 60g sunflower seeds
- 1 sliced kiwi
- 1 sliced orange

Directions:

1. In a bowl, whisk together olive oil, salt, lemon juice, and pepper. Toss the flank steak in this mixture and let it marinate, covered in the fridge, for 30 minutes up to overnight.
2. Preheat your air fryer to 165°C (325°F).
3. Place the marinated flank steak in the greased frying basket of your air fryer.
4. Air Fry for 18-20 minutes until the steak reaches your desired doneness, flipping it once during cooking. Let it rest for 5 minutes before slicing it thinly against the grain.
5. In a salad bowl, whisk together balsamic vinaigrette and Dijon mustard. Stir in arugula, and season with salt and pepper.
6. Divide the dressed arugula mixture between 4 serving bowls.
7. Top each salad with blue cheese, sliced red onion, pecan pieces, sunflower seeds, sliced strawberries, kiwi, orange, and the sliced steak.
8. Serve immediately.

Cal-mex Chimichangas

Servings: 4

Cooking Time: 30 Minutes

Ingredients:

- 1 can diced tomatoes with chiles
- 120g shredded cheddar
- 60g chopped onions
- 2 garlic cloves, minced
- 450g ground beef
- 2 tablespoons taco seasoning
- Salt and pepper to taste
- 4 flour tortillas
- 120ml Pico de Gallo
- Olive oil for cooking
- Cooking oil spray

Directions:

1. Warm the olive oil in a skillet over medium heat, and sauté the onions and minced garlic for 3 minutes or until fragrant.
2. Add the ground beef, taco seasoning, salt, and pepper. Stir and break up the beef with a spoon. Cook for 3-4 minutes or until it is browned.
3. Stir in the diced tomatoes with chiles.
4. Scoop 120ml (½ cup) of the beef mixture onto each tortilla.
5. Form chimichangas by folding the sides of the tortilla into the middle, then roll up from the bottom. Use a toothpick to secure the chimichanga.
6. Preheat your air fryer to 200°C (400°F).
7. Lightly spray the chimichangas with cooking oil.
8. Place the first batch in the air fryer basket and bake for 8 minutes.
9. Transfer the cooked chimichangas to a serving dish and top them with shredded cheese and Pico de Gallo.

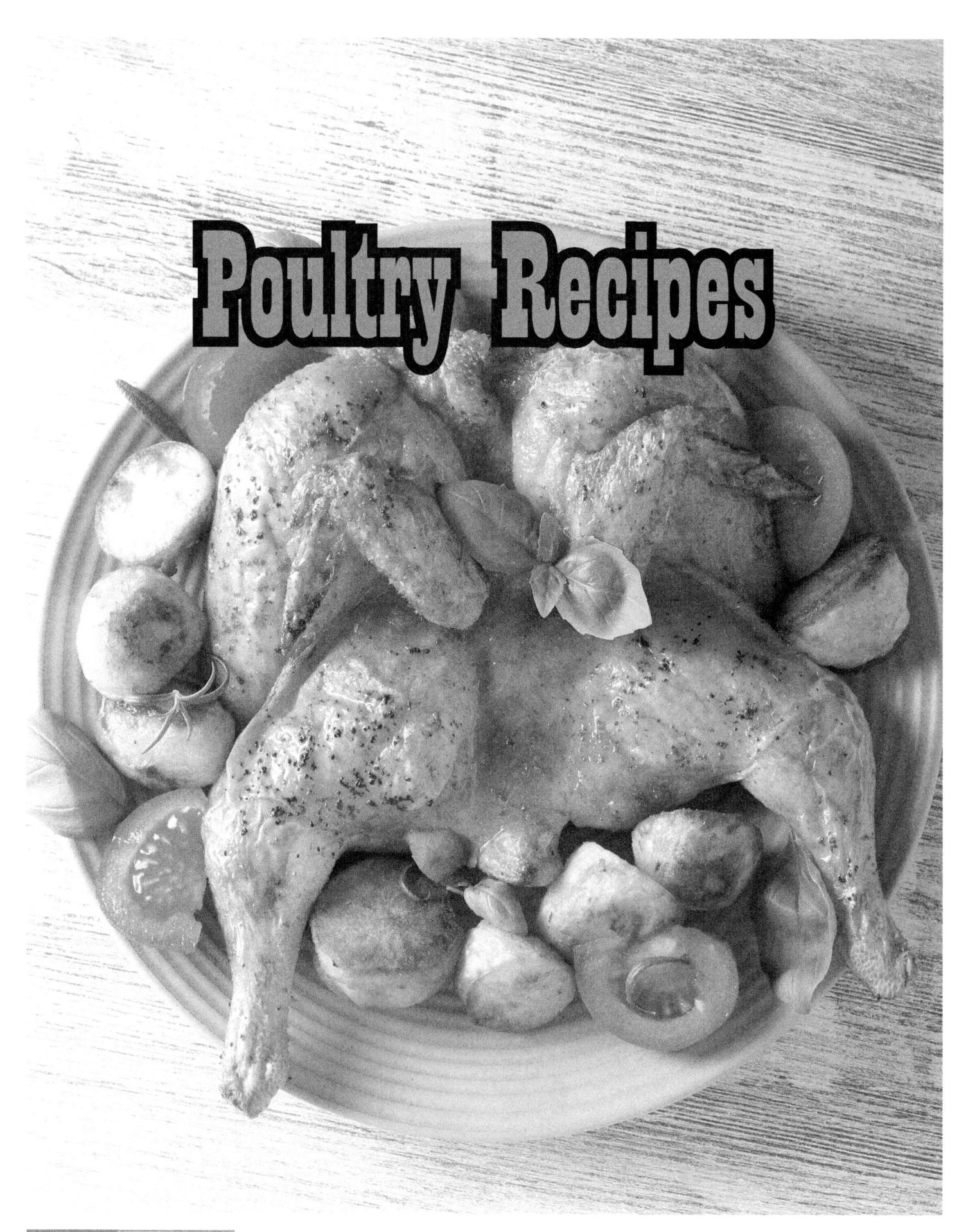

Poultry Recipes

Poultry Recipes

Harissa Chicken Wings

Servings: 4

Cooking Time: 25 Minutes

Ingredients:

- 8 whole chicken wings
- 1 tsp garlic powder
- ¼ tsp dried oregano
- 1 tbsp harissa seasoning

Directions:

1. Preheat the air fryer to 200°C (392°F).
2. Season the wings with garlic powder, harissa seasoning, and dried oregano.
3. Place the seasoned wings in the greased frying basket, and lightly spray them with cooking oil.
4. Air fry for 10 minutes, then shake the basket to ensure even cooking.
5. Continue to air fry for an additional 5-7 minutes or until the wings are golden and crispy.
6. Serve the harissa chicken wings while still warm. Enjoy!

Chicken Strips

Servings: 4

Cooking Time: 8 Minutes

Ingredients:

- 450g chicken tenders
- Marinade:
- 60ml olive oil
- 30ml water
- 30ml honey
- 30ml white vinegar
- 1/2 teaspoon salt
- 1/2 teaspoon crushed red pepper
- 1 teaspoon garlic powder
- 1 teaspoon onion powder
- 1/2 teaspoon paprika

Directions:

1. Combine all the marinade ingredients and mix well.
2. Add the chicken tenders and stir to coat. Cover tightly and let marinate in the refrigerator for 30 minutes.
3. Remove the tenders from the marinade and place them in a single layer in the air fryer basket.
4. Cook at 200°C (390°F) for 3 minutes. Turn the tenders over and cook for 5 minutes longer or until the chicken is cooked through, and the juices run clear.
5. Repeat step 4 to cook the remaining tenders.

Garlic Chicken

Servings: 4

Cooking Time: 30 Minutes

Ingredients:

- 4 bone-in, skinless chicken thighs
- 15 ml olive oil
- 15 ml lemon juice
- 45 ml cornstarch
- 5 ml dried sage
- Black pepper to taste
- 20 garlic cloves, unpeeled

Directions:

1. Preheat the air fryer to 190°C (370°F).
2. Brush the chicken thighs with olive oil and lemon juice. Then, sprinkle with cornstarch, dried sage, and black pepper.
3. Place the chicken thighs in the air fryer basket and scatter the unpeeled garlic cloves on top.
4. Roast for 25 minutes or until the garlic is soft, and the chicken is cooked through.
5. Serve and enjoy your Garlic Chicken.

Granny Pesto Chicken Caprese

Servings: 4

Cooking Time: 30 Minutes

Ingredients:

- 30g grated Parmesan cheese
- 115g fresh mozzarella cheese, thinly sliced
- 16 grape tomatoes, halved
- 4 garlic cloves, minced
- 5ml olive oil
- Salt and pepper to taste
- 4 chicken cutlets
- 15ml prepared pesto
- 1 large egg, beaten
- 60g bread crumbs
- 10ml Italian seasoning
- 5ml balsamic vinegar
- 30g chopped fresh basil

Directions:

1. Preheat the air fryer to 200°C (400°F).
2. In a bowl, coat the grape tomatoes with minced garlic, olive oil, salt, and pepper. Air fry for 5 minutes, shaking the basket twice. Set aside when they are soft.
3. Place the chicken cutlets between two sheets of parchment paper and use a meat mallet to pound them to a 6mm (¼-inch) thickness. Season both sides with salt and pepper.
4. Spread an even coat of pesto on each chicken cutlet.
5. Put the beaten egg in a shallow bowl. In a second shallow bowl, mix the bread crumbs, Italian seasoning, and grated Parmesan cheese.
6. Dip each chicken cutlet in the beaten egg, ensuring it's coated, and then coat it with the breadcrumb mixture. Press the crumbs onto the chicken to make them adhere.
7. Place the chicken cutlets in the greased air fryer basket. Air fry the chicken for 6-8 minutes, flipping once, until they turn golden brown and are cooked through.
8. Put 25g of mozzarella cheese and ¼ of the air-fried tomatoes on top of each chicken cutlet.
9. Once all the cutlets are cooked, return them to the air fryer basket and melt the cheese for 2 minutes.
10. Remove the chicken from the air fryer, drizzle with balsamic vinegar, and sprinkle chopped fresh basil on top.

Farmer's Fried Chicken

Servings: 4

Cooking Time: 55 Minutes

Ingredients:

- 1.36 kg whole chicken, cut into breasts, drumsticks, and thighs
- 475g flour
- 4 tsp salt
- 4 tsp dried basil
- 4 tsp dried thyme
- 2 tsp dried shallot powder
- 2 tsp smoked paprika
- 1 tsp mustard powder
- 1 tsp celery salt
- 240ml kefir
- 60ml honey

Directions:

1. Preheat the air fryer to 190°C.
2. In a bowl, combine the flour, salt, basil, thyme, shallot, paprika, mustard powder, and celery salt. Pour the mixture into a glass jar for dredging.
3. Mix the kefir and honey in a large bowl, then add the chicken pieces. Stir to coat the chicken thoroughly and marinate for 15 minutes at room temperature.
4. Remove the chicken from the kefir mixture, allowing any excess to drip off. Discard the remaining kefir mixture.
5. Place 160g of the flour mixture onto a plate. Dredge each piece of chicken in the flour mixture, shaking gently to remove excess flour. Place the coated chicken pieces on a wire rack for 10 minutes.
6. Line the air fryer basket with round parchment paper with holes punched in it. Arrange the chicken pieces in a single layer and spray them with cooking oil.
7. Air Fry for 18-25 minutes, flipping the chicken pieces once around the 10-minute mark, until they are crispy and cooked through.
8. Serve the Farmer's Fried Chicken hot and enjoy!

Chicken Chunks

Servings: 4

Cooking Time: 10 Minutes

Ingredients:

- 450g chicken tenders, cut into large chunks (about 3.8cm)
- Salt and pepper, to taste
- 120g cornstarch
- 2 eggs, beaten
- 85g panko breadcrumbs
- Oil for misting or cooking spray

Directions:

1. Season the chicken chunks to your liking with salt and pepper.
2. Dip the chicken chunks in cornstarch. Then dip them in the beaten egg, allowing excess to drip off. Finally, roll the chunks in panko breadcrumbs to coat them well.
3. Spray all sides of the chicken chunks with oil or cooking spray.
4. Place the chicken in the air fryer basket in a single layer and cook at 200°C (390°F) for 5 minutes. Spray with oil, then turn the chunks over and spray the other side.
5. Cook for an additional 5 minutes or until the chicken juices run clear, and the outside is golden brown.
6. Repeat steps 4 and 5 to cook the remaining chicken.

Crunchy Chicken Strips

Servings: 4

Cooking Time: 40 Minutes

Ingredients:

- 1 chicken breast, sliced into strips
- 15g grated Parmesan cheese
- 100g breadcrumbs
- 1 tbsp chicken seasoning
- 2 eggs, beaten
- Salt and pepper to taste

Directions:

1. Preheat the air fryer to 175°C.
2. Mix the breadcrumbs, Parmesan cheese, chicken seasoning, salt, and pepper in a mixing bowl.
3. Coat the chicken with the crumb mixture, then dip in the beaten eggs. Finally, coat again with the dry ingredients.
4. Arrange the coated chicken pieces on the greased frying basket and Air Fry for 15 minutes.
5. Turn over halfway through cooking and cook for another 15 minutes.
6. Serve immediately.

Buttery Chicken Legs

Servings: 4

Cooking Time: 50 Minutes

Ingredients:

- 5ml baking powder
- 5ml dried mustard
- 5ml smoked paprika
- 5ml garlic powder
- 5ml dried thyme
- Salt and pepper to taste
- 680 grams chicken legs
- 45ml butter, melted

Directions:

1. Preheat your air fryer to 190°C (370°F).
2. In a bowl, combine all the ingredients, except for the melted butter, until the chicken legs are well coated.
3. Place the chicken legs in the greased frying basket of the air fryer.
4. Air fry for 18 minutes, flipping the chicken legs once and brushing them with melted butter on both sides during cooking.
5. Transfer the cooked chicken legs to a serving plate and let them rest for 5 minutes before serving.

Coconut Chicken With Apricot-ginger Sauce

Servings: 4

Cooking Time: 8 Minutes Per Batch

Ingredients:

- 680g boneless, skinless chicken tenders, cut in large chunks (about 3cm)
- Salt and pepper
- 125g cornstarch
- 2 eggs
- 15ml milk
- 180g shredded coconut (see below)
- Oil for misting or cooking spray
- Apricot-Ginger Sauce:
- 125ml apricot preserves
- 30ml white vinegar
- 1g ground ginger
- 1g low-sodium soy sauce
- 10g white or yellow onion, grated or finely minced

Directions:

1. Mix all ingredients for the Apricot-Ginger Sauce well and let it sit for flavors to blend while you cook the chicken.
2. Season chicken chunks with salt and pepper to taste.
3. Place cornstarch in a shallow dish.
4. In another shallow dish, beat together eggs and milk.
5. Place coconut in a third shallow dish. (If also using panko breadcrumbs, as suggested below, stir them to mix well.)
6. Spray the air fryer basket with oil or cooking spray.
7. Dip each chicken chunk into cornstarch, shake off excess, and dip in the egg mixture.
8. Shake off excess egg mixture and roll lightly in coconut or coconut mixture. Spray with oil.
9. Place coated chicken chunks in the air fryer basket in a single layer, close together but without sides touching.
10. Cook at 180°C for 4 minutes, stop, and turn chunks over.
11. Cook an additional 4 minutes or until chicken is done inside and coating is crispy brown.
12. Repeat steps 9 through 11 to cook remaining chicken chunks.

Chicken Flautas

Servings: 6

Cooking Time: 8 Minutes

Ingredients:

- 6 tablespoons whipped cream cheese
- 150g shredded cooked chicken
- 6 tablespoons mild pico de gallo salsa
- 75g shredded Mexican cheese
- 0.5 teaspoon taco seasoning
- Six 20cm flour tortillas
- 100g shredded lettuce
- 50g guacamole

Directions:

1. Preheat the air fryer to 190°C (370°F).
2. In a large bowl, mix the cream cheese, shredded chicken, salsa, shredded cheese, and taco seasoning until well combined.
3. Lay the tortillas on a flat surface. Divide the cheese-and-chicken mixture into 6 equal portions and place the mixture in the center of each tortilla, spreading it evenly, leaving about 2.5cm from the edge of the tortilla.
4. Spray the air fryer basket with olive oil spray. Roll up the flautas and place them edge side down into the basket. Lightly mist the top of the flautas with olive oil spray.
5. Repeat until the air fryer basket is full. You may need to cook these in batches, depending on the size of your air fryer.
6. Cook for 7 minutes, or until the outer edges are browned.
7. Remove from the air fryer basket and serve warm over a bed of shredded lettuce with guacamole on top.

Chicken Cordon Bleu

Servings: 4

Cooking Time: 20 Minutes

Ingredients:

- 4 small boneless, skinless chicken breasts
- Salt and pepper, to taste
- 4 slices of deli ham
- 4 slices of deli Swiss cheese (approximately 7.5 to 10 cm square)
- 2 tablespoons olive oil
- 2 teaspoons dried marjoram
- ¼ teaspoon paprika

Directions:

1. Begin by carefully slicing each chicken breast horizontally, leaving one edge intact.
2. Lay the chicken breasts open flat and season them with salt and pepper to your liking.
3. On top of each chicken breast, place a slice of ham.
4. Cut the cheese slices in half and position one-half on each chicken breast, reserving the remaining halves for later use.
5. Carefully roll up the chicken breasts to enclose the cheese and ham, securing them in place with toothpicks.
6. In a small bowl, combine the olive oil, dried marjoram, and paprika. Mix well and rub this mixture evenly over the outsides of the chicken breasts.
7. Place the prepared chicken in the air fryer basket and cook at 180°C (360°F) for approximately 20 minutes or until the chicken is thoroughly cooked, and the juices run clear.
8. Remove all toothpicks from the chicken breasts. To avoid any burns, transfer the chicken breasts to a plate to remove the toothpicks safely, and then return them immediately to the air fryer basket.
9. Lastly, add half a cheese slice on top of each chicken breast, and cook for an additional minute or until the cheese has melted and is slightly bubbly.

Irresistible Cheesy Chicken Sticks

Servings: 2

Cooking Time: 30 Minutes

Ingredients:

- 6 mozzarella sticks
- 120g flour
- 2 eggs, beaten
- 450g ground chicken
- 150g breadcrumbs
- 1/4 tsp crushed chilis
- 1/4 tsp cayenne pepper
- 1/2 tsp garlic powder
- 1/4 tsp shallot powder
- 1/2 tsp dried oregano

Directions:

1. Preheat the air fryer to 200°C (390°F).
2. In a bowl, combine crushed chilis, cayenne pepper, garlic powder, shallot powder, and dried oregano. Add the ground chicken and mix thoroughly until evenly combined.
3. In another mixing bowl, beat the eggs until they are fluffy and well-combined.
4. Pour the beaten eggs, flour, and breadcrumbs into three separate bowls.
5. Roll each mozzarella stick in the flour, then dip it in the beaten eggs.
6. Using your hands, wrap each stick in a thin layer of the chicken mixture.
7. Finally, coat the sticks in the breadcrumbs, ensuring they are evenly covered.
8. Place the coated sticks in the greased air fryer frying basket.
9. Air Fry for 18-20 minutes, turning them once during cooking to ensure even crisping.
10. Serve your Irresistible Cheesy Chicken Sticks while hot.

Chicago-style Turkey Meatballs

Servings: 6

Cooking Time: 15 Minutes

Ingredients:

- 450 grams ground turkey
- 15ml orange juice
- Salt and pepper to taste
- 2.5ml smoked paprika
- 2.5ml chili powder
- 5ml cumin powder
- 1/4 red bell pepper, diced
- 1 diced jalapeño pepper
- 2 garlic cloves, minced

Directions:

1. Preheat your air fryer to 200°C (400°F).
2. In a large bowl, combine all of the ingredients.
3. Shape the mixture into meatballs.
4. Transfer the meatballs into the greased air fryer frying basket.
5. Air fry the meatballs for 4 minutes, then flip them.
6. Air fry for an additional 3 minutes or until the meatballs are cooked through.
7. Serve your Chicago-Style Turkey Meatballs immediately.

Cajun Fried Chicken

Servings: 3

Cooking Time: 35 Minutes

Ingredients:

- 240ml Cajun seasoning
- 2.5ml mango powder
- 6 chicken legs, bone-in

Directions:

1. Preheat your air fryer to 180°C (360°F).
2. Place half of the Cajun seasoning and 180ml (3/4 cup) of water in a bowl and mix well to dissolve any lumps.
3. In a shallow bowl, combine the remaining Cajun seasoning and mango powder, stirring to combine.
4. Dip each chicken leg in the batter mixture, then coat it in the mango seasoning.
5. Lightly spritz the chicken legs with cooking spray to help with browning.
6. Place the coated chicken legs in the air fryer.
7. Air fry the chicken for 14-16 minutes, turning them once during cooking, until the chicken is cooked through, and the coating is brown.
8. Serve and enjoy your Cajun Fried Chicken!

Gruyère Asparagus & Chicken Quiche

Servings: 4

Cooking Time: 30 Minutes

Ingredients:

- 1 grilled chicken breast, diced
- 60g shredded Gruyère cheese
- 1 premade pie crust
- 2 eggs, beaten
- 60ml milk
- Salt and pepper to taste
- 225g asparagus, sliced
- 1 lemon, zested

Directions:

1. Preheat the air fryer to 180°C (360°F).
2. Carefully press the pie crust into a baking dish, trimming the edges. Prick the dough with a fork a few times.
3. In a mixing bowl, combine the beaten eggs, milk, sliced asparagus, salt, pepper, diced chicken, lemon zest, and half of the Gruyère cheese. Stir until the mixture is well blended.
4. Pour the mixture into the pie crust.
5. Bake in the air fryer for 15 minutes.
6. Sprinkle the remaining Gruyère cheese on top of the quiche filling.
7. Continue to bake for an additional 5 minutes until the quiche is golden brown.
8. Remove from the air fryer and allow it to cool for a few minutes before cutting.
9. Serve sliced and enjoy your Gruyère Asparagus & Chicken Quiche!

Cal-mex Turkey Patties

Servings: 4

Cooking Time: 30 Minutes

Ingredients:

- 40 grams crushed corn tortilla chips
- 40 grams grated American cheese
- 1 egg, beaten
- 60ml salsa
- Salt and pepper to taste
- 450 grams ground turkey
- 15ml olive oil
- 5 grams chili powder

Directions:

1. Preheat your air fryer to 165°C (330°F).
2. In a bowl, mix together the beaten egg, crushed corn tortilla chips, salsa, grated American cheese, salt, and pepper.
3. Add the ground turkey to the mixture and gently combine using your hands until just mixed.
4. Divide the meat mixture into 4 equal portions and shape them into patties about 1.25 centimeters (½ inch) thick.
5. Brush the patties with olive oil and sprinkle them with chili powder.
6. Air fry the patties for 14-16 minutes, flipping them once during cooking, until they are cooked through and golden brown.
7. Serve your Cal-Mex Turkey Patties and enjoy!

Creole Chicken Drumettes

Servings: 4

Cooking Time: 50 Minutes

Ingredients:

- 450g chicken drumettes
- 65g flour
- 120ml double cream
- 120ml sour cream
- 65g breadcrumbs
- 15g Creole seasoning
- 30g melted butter

Directions:

1. Preheat the air fryer to 190°C.
2. Combine chicken drumettes and flour in a bowl. Shake away excess flour and set aside.
3. Mix the double cream and sour cream in a bowl.
4. In another bowl, combine breadcrumbs and Creole seasoning.
5. Dip floured drumettes in the cream mixture, then dredge them in the breadcrumb mixture.
6. Place the chicken drumettes in the greased frying basket of the air fryer.
7. Air Fry for 20 minutes, tossing once and brushing with melted butter.
8. Let them rest for a few minutes on a plate, and then serve your Creole Chicken Drumettes. Enjoy!

Chicken Flatbread Pizza With Spinach

Servings: 1

Cooking Time: 15 Minutes

Ingredients:

- 65g cooked chicken breast, cubed
- 30g grated mozzarella
- 1 whole-wheat pita
- 15ml olive oil
- 1 garlic clove, minced
- 0.25 tsp red pepper flakes
- 65g kale
- 15g sliced red onion

Directions:

1. Preheat the air fryer to 190°C (380°F).
2. Lightly brush the top of the pita with olive oil and top with the minced garlic, red pepper flakes, kale, red onion slices, cubed chicken, and mozzarella.
3. Place the pizza into the air fryer basket and cook for 7 minutes or until the cheese is melted and the edges are crispy.
4. Serve and enjoy your Chicken Flatbread Pizza with Spinach!

Chicken Cordon Bleu Patties

Servings: 4

Cooking Time: 30 Minutes

Ingredients:

- 35g grated Fontina cheese
- 45ml milk
- 35g bread crumbs
- 1 egg, beaten
- 2.5ml dried parsley
- Salt and pepper, to taste
- 570g ground chicken
- 30g finely chopped ham

Directions:

1. Preheat the air fryer to 175°C (350°F).
2. In a bowl, mix together the milk, breadcrumbs, beaten egg, dried parsley, salt, and pepper.
3. Add the ground chicken to the mixture and gently combine until just mixed.
4. Divide the mixture into 8 portions and shape them into thin patties. Place them on a sheet of waxed paper.
5. On 4 of the patties, top each with chopped ham and Fontina cheese. Place another patty on top of each to create a sandwich, then gently pinch the edges together to seal, ensuring none of the ham or cheese is exposed.
6. Arrange the patties in the greased air fryer basket.
7. Air fry for 14-16 minutes or until the patties are cooked through and have a golden-brown exterior.
8. Serve and enjoy your Chicken Cordon Bleu Patties!

Crispy Chicken Parmesan

Servings: 4

Cooking Time: 12 Minutes

Ingredients:

- 4 skinless, boneless chicken breasts, pounded thin to ¼-inch thickness
- 1 teaspoon salt, divided
- ½ teaspoon black pepper, divided
- 120g flour
- 2 eggs
- 70g panko breadcrumbs
- ½ teaspoon dried oregano
- 50g grated Parmesan cheese

Directions:

1. Pat the chicken breasts with a paper towel. Season the chicken with ½ teaspoon of the salt and ¼ teaspoon of the pepper.
2. In a medium bowl, place the flour.
3. In a second bowl, whisk the eggs.
4. In a third bowl, place the breadcrumbs, oregano, cheese, and the remaining ½ teaspoon of salt and ¼ teaspoon of pepper.
5. Dredge the chicken in the flour and shake off the excess. Dip the chicken into the eggs and then into the breadcrumb mixture. Set the chicken on a plate and repeat with the remaining chicken pieces.
6. Preheat the air fryer to 180°C.
7. Place the chicken in the air fryer basket and spray liberally with cooking spray. Cook for 8 minutes, turn the chicken breasts over, and cook for another 4 minutes. When golden brown, check for an internal temperature of 74°C.

Desserts And Sweets

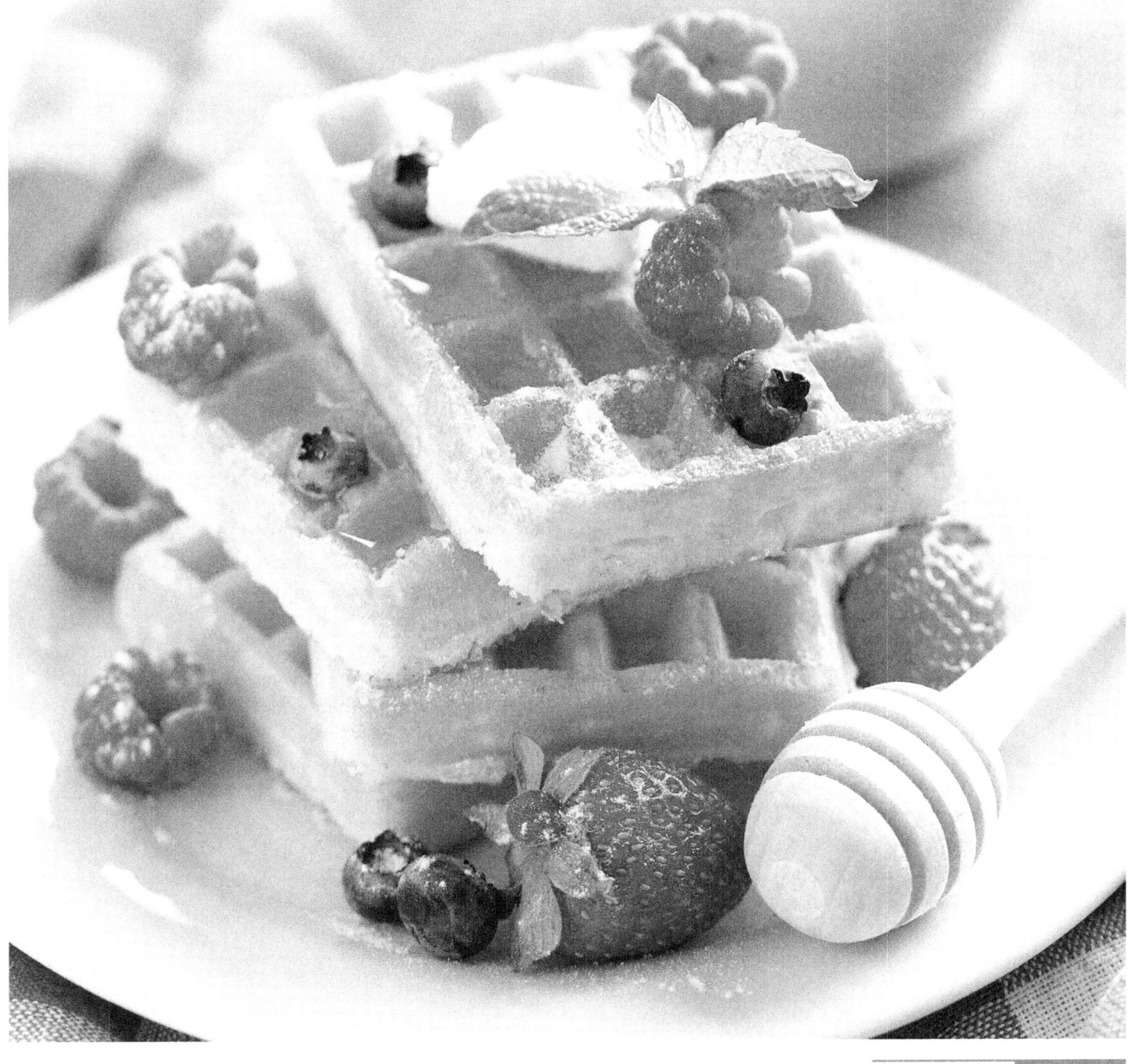

Desserts And Sweets

Caramel Apple Crumble

Servings: 6

Cooking Time: 50 Minutes

Ingredients:

- 4 apples, peeled and thinly sliced
- 30 grams sugar
- 15 grams flour
- 2 grams ground cinnamon
- 0.25 grams ground allspice
- A healthy pinch of ground nutmeg
- 10 caramel squares, cut into small pieces
- Crumble Topping:
- 75 grams rolled oats
- 60 grams sugar
- 45 grams flour
- 1 gram ground cinnamon
- 85 grams butter, melted

Directions:

1. Preheat the air fryer to 165°C (330°F).
2. Combine the apples, sugar, flour, and spices in a large bowl and toss to coat. Add the caramel pieces and mix well.
3. Pour the apple mixture into a 1-quart round baking dish that will fit in your air fryer basket (15 cm diameter).
4. To make the crumble topping, combine the rolled oats, sugar, flour, and ground cinnamon in a small bowl. Add the melted butter and mix well.
5. Top the apples with the crumble mixture. Cover the entire dish with aluminum foil and transfer the dish to the air fryer basket, lowering the dish into the basket using a sling made of aluminum foil (fold a piece of aluminum foil into a strip about 5 cm wide by 60 cm long). Fold the ends of the aluminum foil over the top of the dish before returning the basket to the air fryer.
6. Air-fry at 165°C (330°F) for 25 minutes. Remove the aluminum foil and continue to air-fry for another 25 minutes.
7. Serve the crumble warm with whipped cream or vanilla ice cream, if desired.

Mango-chocolate Custard

Servings: 4

Cooking Time: 40 Minutes

Ingredients:

- 4 egg yolks
- 2 tbsp granulated sugar
- 1/8 tsp almond extract
- 360ml half-and-half
- 135g chocolate chips
- 1 mango, pureed
- 1 mango, chopped
- 1 tsp fresh mint, chopped

Directions:

1. In a bowl, beat the egg yolks, granulated sugar, and almond extract. Set aside.
2. Place the half-and-half in a saucepan over low heat and bring it to a low simmer. Whisk a spoonful of the heated half-and-half into the egg mixture, then slowly whisk the egg mixture into the saucepan.
3. Stir in the chocolate chips and mango puree, and cook for 10 minutes or until the chocolate melts.
4. Divide the custard mixture between 4 ramekins.
5. Preheat the oven to 180°C (350°F). Place the ramekins in an ovenproof dish or a baking pan and fill the dish with hot water until it reaches halfway up the sides of the ramekins.
6. Bake for 6-8 minutes until the custard is set but still slightly jiggly in the center.
7. Remove from the oven and let cool on a cooling rack for 15 minutes, then cover and refrigerate for at least 2 hours or up to 2 days.
8. Serve the custard with chopped mangoes and mint on top.

Chewy Coconut Cake

Servings: 6

Cooking Time: 18-22 Minutes

Ingredients:

- 100 grams plus 2.5 tablespoons All-purpose flour
- 3/4 teaspoon Baking powder
- 1/8 teaspoon Table salt
- 85 grams (1 stick minus 1/2 tablespoon) Butter, at room temperature
- 85 grams plus 1 tablespoon Granulated white sugar
- 75 grams Packed light brown sugar
- 75 grams Pasteurized egg substitute, such as Egg Beaters
- 10 milliliters Vanilla extract
- 40 grams Unsweetened shredded coconut
- Baking spray

Directions:

1. Preheat the air fryer to 160°C (or 165°C if that's the closest setting).
2. Mix the flour, baking powder, and salt in a small bowl until well combined.
3. Using an electric hand mixer at medium speed, beat the butter, granulated white sugar, and brown sugar in a medium bowl until creamy and smooth, about 3 minutes, occasionally scraping down the inside of the bowl. Beat in the egg substitute or egg and vanilla until smooth.
4. Scrape down and remove the beaters. Fold in the flour mixture with a rubber spatula just until all the flour is moistened. Fold in the coconut until the mixture is a uniform color.
5. Use the baking spray to generously coat the inside of a 15 cm (6-inch) round cake pan for a small batch, an 18 cm (7-inch) round cake pan for a medium batch, or a 20 cm (8-inch) round cake pan for a large batch. Scrape and spread the batter into the pan, smoothing the batter out to an even layer.
6. Set the pan in the basket and air-fry for 18 minutes for a 15 cm (6-inch) layer, 20 minutes for an 18 cm (7-inch) layer, or 22 minutes for a 20 cm (8-inch) layer, or until the cake is well browned and set even if there's a little soft give right at the center. Start checking it at the 16-minute mark to know where you are.
7. Use hot pads or silicone baking mitts to transfer the cake pan to a wire rack. Cool for at least 1 hour or up to 4 hours. Use a nonstick-safe knife to slice the cake into wedges right in the pan, lifting them out one by one.
8. Enjoy your Chewy Coconut Cake!

Mixed Berry Pie

Servings: 4

Cooking Time: 25 Minutes

Ingredients:

- 150g blackberries, cut into thirds
- 60g sugar
- 30ml cornstarch
- 1.25ml vanilla extract
- 1.25ml peppermint extract
- 1.25ml lemon zest
- 150g sliced strawberries
- 150g raspberries
- 1 refrigerated piecrust
- 1 large egg

Directions:

1. Mix the sugar, cornstarch, vanilla extract, peppermint extract, and lemon zest in a bowl. Gently toss in all the berries until they are combined.
2. Pour the berry mixture into a greased baking dish.
3. On a clean workspace, lay out the piecrust and cut it into a 18cm diameter round.
4. Cover the baking dish with the round piecrust and crimp the edges. Use a knife to cut 4 slits in the top crust to allow steam to vent.
5. Beat 1 egg and 15ml of water to make an egg wash. Brush the egg wash over the crust.
6. Preheat the air fryer to 180°C (350°F). Place the baking dish into the frying basket.
7. Bake for 15 minutes or until the crust is golden and the berries are bubbling through the vents.
8. Remove the pie from the air fryer and let it cool for 15 minutes.
9. Serve the mixed berry pie warm.

Molten Chocolate Almond Cakes

Servings: 3

Cooking Time: 13 Minutes

Ingredients:

- Butter and flour for the ramekins
- 115g bittersweet chocolate, chopped
- 115g unsalted butter (1 stick)
- 2 eggs
- 2 egg yolks
- 60g sugar
- 2.5ml pure vanilla extract or almond extract
- 15ml all-purpose flour
- 45g ground almonds
- 8 to 12 semisweet chocolate discs (or 4 chunks of chocolate)
- Cocoa powder or powdered sugar, for dusting
- Toasted almonds, coarsely chopped

Directions:

1. Butter and flour three (170ml) ramekins. Butter the ramekins and then coat the butter with flour by shaking it around in the ramekin and dumping out any excess.
2. Melt the chocolate and butter together, either in the microwave or in a double boiler.
3. In a separate bowl, beat the eggs, egg yolks, and sugar together until light and smooth. Add the vanilla extract.
4. Whisk the melted chocolate mixture into the egg mixture. Stir in the flour and ground almonds.
5. Preheat the air fryer to 165°C (330°F).
6. Carefully transfer the batter to the buttered ramekins, filling them halfway. Place two or three chocolate discs in the center of the batter and then fill the ramekins to 1.25cm below the top with the remaining batter.
7. Place the ramekins into the air fryer basket and air-fry at 165°C (330°F) for 13 minutes. The sides of the cakes should be set, but the centers should be slightly soft. If you prefer the cakes a little less molten, air-fry for 14 minutes and let the cakes sit for 4 minutes.
8. Run a butter knife around the edge of the ramekins and invert the cakes onto a plate. Lift the ramekin off the plate slowly and carefully so that the cake doesn't break.
9. Dust the cakes with cocoa powder or powdered sugar and serve with a scoop of ice cream and some coarsely chopped toasted almonds.

Honey-roasted Mixed Nuts

Servings: 8

Cooking Time: 15 Minutes

Ingredients:

- 60 grams raw, shelled pistachios
- 60 grams raw almonds
- 125 grams raw walnuts
- 30 milliliters filtered water
- 30 milliliters honey
- 15 milliliters vegetable oil
- 30 grams sugar
- 1/2 teaspoon salt

Directions:

1. Preheat the air fryer to 150°C (300°F).
2. Lightly spray an air-fryer-safe pan with olive oil. Place the pistachios, almonds, and walnuts inside the pan, and then place the pan inside the air fryer basket.
3. Cook for 15 minutes, shaking the basket every 5 minutes to rotate the nuts for even roasting.
4. While the nuts are roasting, in a small pan, boil the water and stir in the honey and oil. Continue to stir while cooking until the water begins to evaporate, and a thick syrup is formed. The syrup should stick to the back of a wooden spoon when mixed. Turn off the heat.
5. Remove the nuts from the air fryer when cooking is completed, and spoon them into the stovetop pan with the honey syrup. Use a spatula to coat the nuts with the honey syrup.
6. Line a baking sheet with parchment paper and spoon the coated nuts onto the sheet.
7. Lightly sprinkle the sugar and salt over the nuts.
8. Let the nuts cool in the refrigerator for at least 2 hours until the honey and sugar have hardened.
9. Once the honey and sugar have set, store the honey-roasted mixed nuts in an airtight container in the refrigerator.

Baked Apple

Servings: 6

Cooking Time: 20 Minutes

Ingredients:

- 3 small Honey Crisp or other baking apples
- 3 tablespoons maple syrup
- 3 tablespoons chopped pecans
- 1 tablespoon firm butter, cut into 6 pieces

Directions:

1. Pour 120 ml (1/2 cup) of water into the drawer of the air fryer.
2. Thoroughly wash and dry the apples.
3. Cut the apples in half and remove the core and a little bit of the flesh to create a hollow cavity for the pecans.
4. Place the apple halves in the air fryer basket, with the cut side facing up.
5. Spoon 7.5 ml (1.5 teaspoons) of chopped pecans into each apple's cavity.
6. Drizzle 7.5 ml (1/2 tablespoon) of maple syrup over the pecans inside each apple.
7. Top each apple half with 2.5 ml (1/2 teaspoon) of butter.
8. Cook in the air fryer at 180°C (360°F) for 20 minutes or until the apples are tender.

Cinnamon Canned Biscuit Donuts

Servings: 4

Cooking Time: 25 Minutes

Ingredients:

- 1 can jumbo biscuits
- 200 grams (1 cup) cinnamon sugar

Directions:

1. Preheat your air fryer to 180°C (360°F).
2. Divide the biscuit dough into 8 biscuits and place them on a flat work surface.
3. Use a small cookie cutter to cut a small circle in the center of each biscuit, creating the donut shape.
4. Place a batch of 4 donuts in the air fryer basket, ensuring they have enough space between them.
5. Spray the donuts with a light coat of cooking oil to promote browning.
6. Bake in the air fryer at 180°C (360°F) for 8 minutes, flipping them once during cooking to ensure even browning.
7. While the donuts are still warm, drizzle them generously with the cinnamon sugar mixture.
8. Repeat the process with the remaining batch of donuts.
9. Serve your Cinnamon Canned Biscuit Donuts and enjoy!

Fast Brownies

Servings: 4

Cooking Time: 25 Minutes

Ingredients:

- 60 grams flour
- 10 grams cocoa powder
- 75 grams granulated sugar
- 1/4 teaspoon baking soda
- 40 grams butter, melted
- 1 egg
- 1/4 teaspoon salt
- 75 grams chocolate chips
- 30 grams chopped hazelnuts
- 10 grams powdered sugar
- 5 ml (1 teaspoon) vanilla extract

Directions:

1. Preheat your air fryer to 180°C (350°F).
2. In a bowl, combine all the ingredients, except for the chocolate chips, hazelnuts, and powdered sugar.
3. Fold in the chocolate chips and chopped hazelnuts.
4. Press the mixture into a greased cake pan.
5. Place the cake pan in the air fryer basket.
6. Bake the brownies in the air fryer for 12 minutes.
7. Allow the brownies to cool for 10 minutes before slicing them into 9 brownies.
8. Scatter powdered sugar over the brownies before serving.

Black And Blue Clafoutis

Servings: 2

Cooking Time: 15 Minutes

Ingredients:

- 6-inch pie pan
- 3 large eggs
- 120 grams sugar
- 1 teaspoon vanilla extract
- 28 grams butter, melted
- 240 ml milk
- 60 grams all-purpose flour*
- 120 grams blackberries
- 120 grams blueberries
- 2 tablespoons icing sugar (confectioners' sugar)

Directions:

1. Preheat the air fryer to 160°C (320°F).
2. In a bowl, combine the eggs and sugar, then whisk vigorously until the mixture is smooth, lighter in color, and well combined.
3. Add the vanilla extract, melted butter, and milk to the egg-sugar mixture and whisk together thoroughly.
4. Gradually add the all-purpose flour and whisk just until no lumps or streaks of white remain.
5. Scatter half of the blueberries and blackberries in a greased 6-inch pie pan or cake pan.
6. Pour half of the batter (approximately 300 ml) over the berries.
7. Transfer the tart pan to the air fryer basket. You can use an aluminum foil sling to help with this by taking a long piece of aluminum foil, folding it in half lengthwise twice until it is roughly 66 cm by 5 cm. Place this under the pie dish and hold the ends of the foil to move the pie dish in and out of the air fryer basket. Tuck the ends of the foil beside the pie dish while it cooks in the air fryer.
8. Air-fry at 160°C (320°F) for 15 minutes or until the clafoutis has puffed up and is still slightly jiggly in the center.
9. Remove the clafoutis from the air fryer, invert it onto a plate, and let it cool while you bake the second batch.
10. Serve the clafoutis warm, dusted with icing sugar on top.

Glazed Cherry Turnovers

Servings: 8

Cooking Time: 14 Minutes

Ingredients:

- 2 sheets of frozen puff pastry, thawed
- 1 (595-gram) can of premium cherry pie filling
- 2 teaspoons ground cinnamon
- 1 egg, beaten
- 100 grams sliced almonds
- 125 grams icing sugar (powdered sugar)
- 30 milliliters milk

Directions:

1. Roll a sheet of puff pastry out into a square that is approximately 25 centimeters by 25 centimeters. Cut this large square into quarters.
2. Mix the cherry pie filling and cinnamon together in a bowl. Spoon 60 milliliters (1/4 cup) of the cherry filling into the center of each puff pastry square. Brush the perimeter of the pastry square with the beaten egg. Fold one corner of the puff pastry over the cherry pie filling towards the opposite corner, forming a triangle. Seal the two edges of the pastry together with the tip of a fork, making a design with the tines. Brush the top of the turnovers with the beaten egg and sprinkle sliced almonds over each one. Repeat these steps with the second sheet of puff pastry. You should have eight turnovers at the end.
3. Preheat the air fryer to 190°C (370°F).
4. Air-fry two turnovers at a time for 14 minutes, carefully turning them over halfway through the cooking time.
5. While the turnovers are cooking, make the glaze by whisking the icing sugar and milk together in a small bowl until smooth. Let the glaze sit for a minute so the sugar can absorb the milk. If the consistency is still too thick to drizzle, add a little more milk, a drop at a time, and stir until smooth.
6. Let the cooked cherry turnovers sit for at least 10 minutes. Then drizzle the glaze over each turnover in a zigzag motion. Serve warm or at room temperature.

Apple Dumplings

Servings: 4

Cooking Time: 10 Minutes

Ingredients:

- 4 Small tart apples, preferably McIntosh, peeled and cored
- 60g Granulated white sugar
- 1½ tablespoons Ground cinnamon
- 1 sheet, thawed and cut into four quarters of frozen puff pastry (vegetarian, if a concern)

Directions:

1. Set the apples (former) stem side up on a microwave-safe plate, preferably a glass pie plate. Microwave on high for 3 minutes, or until somewhat tender (but not soft) when poked with the point of a knife. Cool to room temperature, about 30 minutes.
2. Preheat the air fryer to 200°C (400°F).
3. Combine the sugar and cinnamon in a small bowl. Roll the apples in this mixture, coating them completely on their outsides. Also, sprinkle this cinnamon sugar into each hole where the core was.
4. Roll the puff pastry squares into 15 x 15 cm (6 x 6-inch) squares. Slice the corners off each rolled square so that it's sort of like a circle (with four otherwise straight edges, of course). Place an apple in the center of one of these squares and fold it up and all around the apple, sealing it at the top by pressing the pastry together. The apple must be completely sealed in the pastry. Repeat for the remaining apples.
5. Set the pastry-covered apples in the basket with at least 1.25 cm (1/2 inch) between them. Air-fry undisturbed for 10 minutes, or until puffed and golden brown.
6. Use a nonstick-safe spatula, and maybe a flatware tablespoon for balance, to transfer the apples to a wire rack. Cool for at least 5 minutes or up to 15 minutes before serving warm.

Annie's Chocolate Chunk Hazelnut Cookies

Servings: 24

Cooking Time: 12 Minutes

Ingredients:

- 225g butter, softened
- 200g brown sugar
- 100g granulated sugar
- 2 eggs, lightly beaten
- 1½ teaspoons vanilla extract
- 190g all-purpose flour
- 50g rolled oats
- 1 teaspoon baking soda
- ½ teaspoon salt
- 360g chocolate chunks
- 65g toasted chopped hazelnuts

Directions:

1. Cream the butter and sugars together until light and fluffy using a stand mixer or electric hand mixer. Add the eggs and vanilla, and beat until well combined.
2. Combine the flour, rolled oats, baking soda, and salt in a second bowl. Gradually add the dry ingredients to the wet ingredients with a wooden spoon or spatula. Stir in the chocolate chunks and hazelnuts until distributed throughout the dough.
3. Shape the cookies into small balls about the size of golf balls and place them on a baking sheet. Freeze the cookie balls for at least 30 minutes, or package them in as airtight a package as you can and keep them in your freezer.
4. When you're ready for a delicious snack or dessert, preheat the air fryer to 175°C (350°F). Cut a piece of parchment paper to fit the number of cookies you are baking. Place the parchment down in the air fryer basket and place the frozen cookie ball or balls on top (remember to leave room for them to expand).
5. Air-fry the cookies at 175°C (350°F) for 12 minutes, or until they are done to your liking. Let them cool for a few minutes before enjoying your freshly baked cookie.

Fried Twinkies

Servings: 6

Cooking Time: 5 Minutes

Ingredients:

- 2 Large egg white(s)
- 2 tablespoons Water
- 255 grams (about 9 ounces) Ground gingersnap cookie crumbs
- 6 Twinkies
- Vegetable oil spray

Directions:

1. Preheat your air fryer to 200°C (400°F).
2. Set up and fill two shallow soup plates or small pie plates on your counter: one for the egg white(s), whisked with the water until foamy, and one for the gingersnap crumbs.
3. Dip a Twinkie in the egg white(s), turning it to coat on all sides, including the ends. Allow any excess egg white mixture to drip back into the bowl, then place the Twinkie in the crumbs. Roll it to coat on all sides, including the ends, pressing gently to ensure an even coating. Repeat this process for each Twinkie: dip in egg white(s) followed by the crumbs. Lightly coat each prepared Twinkie on all sides with vegetable oil spray. Set them aside and repeat the double-dipping and spraying process for the remaining Twinkies.
4. Place the Twinkies flat side up in the air fryer basket, ensuring there is enough space between them for air circulation. Air-fry for 5 minutes, or until they are browned and crunchy.
5. Use a nonstick-safe spatula to gently transfer the Twinkies to a wire rack. Allow them to cool for at least 10 minutes before serving.

Coconut Macaroons

Servings: 12

Cooking Time: 8 Minutes

Ingredients:

- 160 grams shredded sweetened coconut
- 11 grams flour
- 25 grams sugar
- 1 egg white
- 2.5 ml (1/2 teaspoon) almond extract

Directions:

1. Preheat your air fryer to 165°C (330°F).
2. In a mixing bowl, combine the shredded sweetened coconut, flour, sugar, egg white, and almond extract. Mix all the ingredients together until well combined.
3. Shape the coconut mixture into 12 small balls.
4. Place all 12 macaroons in the air fryer basket. They won't expand, so you can place them close together, but make sure they don't touch.
5. Cook the macaroons in the air fryer at 165°C (330°F) for 8 minutes or until they turn golden brown.
6. Once done, remove the Coconut Macaroons from the air fryer and let them cool slightly.
7. Enjoy your Coconut Macaroons!

Carrot-oat Cake Muffins

Servings: 4

Cooking Time: 20 Minutes

Ingredients:

- 43 grams butter, softened
- 55 grams brown sugar
- 15 ml maple syrup
- 1 egg white
- 2.5 ml vanilla extract
- 80 grams finely grated carrots
- 40 grams oatmeal
- 43 grams flour
- 2.5 ml baking soda
- 20 grams raisins

Directions:

1. Preheat the air fryer to 175°C (350°F).
2. Mix the butter, brown sugar, and maple syrup until smooth, then toss in the egg white, vanilla, and carrots. Whisk well and add the oatmeal, flour, baking soda, and raisins.
3. Divide the mixture between muffin cups.
4. Bake in the fryer for 8-10 minutes.

Mixed Berry Hand Pies

Servings: 4

Cooking Time: 15 Minutes

Ingredients:

- 150g sugar
- 2.5ml ground cinnamon
- 15ml cornstarch
- 150g blueberries
- 150g blackberries
- 150g raspberries, divided
- 5ml water
- 1 package refrigerated pie dough (or your own homemade pie dough)
- 1 egg, beaten

Directions:

1. Combine the sugar, ground cinnamon, and cornstarch in a small saucepan. Add the blueberries, blackberries, and 75g of raspberries. Toss the berries gently to coat them evenly. Add the teaspoon of water to the saucepan and turn the stovetop on to medium-high heat, stirring occasionally. Once the berries break down, release their juice and start to simmer (about 5 minutes), simmer for another couple of minutes and then transfer the mixture to a bowl. Stir in the remaining 75g of raspberries and let it cool.
2. Preheat the air fryer to 190°C (370°F).
3. Cut the pie dough into four 13cm circles and four 15cm circles.
4. Spread the 15cm circles on a flat surface. Divide the berry filling between all four circles. Brush the perimeter of the dough circles with a little water. Place the 13cm circles on top of the filling and press the perimeter of the dough circles together to seal. Roll the edges of the bottom circle up over the top circle to make a crust around the filling. Press a fork around the crust to make decorative indentations and to seal the crust shut. Brush the pies with egg wash and sprinkle a little sugar on top. Poke a small hole in the center of each pie with a paring knife to vent the dough.
5. Air-fry two pies at a time. Brush or spray the air fryer basket with oil and place the pies into the basket. Air-fry for 9 minutes. Turn the pies over and air-fry for another 6 minutes.
6. Serve the hand pies warm or at room temperature.

Chocolate Macaroons

Servings: 16

Cooking Time: 8 Minutes

Ingredients:

- 2 large egg whites, at room temperature
- 1/8 teaspoon table salt
- 120 grams granulated white sugar
- 180 grams unsweetened shredded coconut
- 3 tablespoons unsweetened cocoa powder

Directions:

1. Preheat your air fryer to 190°C (375°F).
2. Using an electric mixer at high speed, beat the egg whites and salt in a medium or large bowl until stiff peaks can be formed when the turned-off beaters are dipped into the mixture.
3. Still working with the mixer at high speed, beat in the granulated white sugar in a slow stream until the meringue is shiny and thick.
4. Scrape down and remove the beaters. Fold in the unsweetened shredded coconut and unsweetened cocoa powder with a rubber spatula until well combined, working carefully to deflate the meringue as little as possible.
5. Scoop up 2 tablespoons of the mixture. Wet your clean hands and roll that little bit of coconut mixture into a ball. Set it aside and continue making more balls: 7 more for a small batch, 15 more for a medium batch, or 23 more for a large one.
6. Line the bottom of the air fryer's basket or the basket attachment with parchment paper. Set the macaroon balls on the parchment with as much air space between them as possible.
7. Air-fry undisturbed for 8 minutes, or until the macaroons are dry, set, and lightly browned.
8. Use a nonstick-safe spatula to transfer the macaroons to a wire rack.
9. Allow the macaroons to cool for at least 10 minutes before serving. Alternatively, you can cool them to room temperature (about 30 minutes) and then store them in a sealed container at room temperature for up to 3 days.

MEASUREMENT CONVERSIONS

BASIC KITCHEN CONVERSIONS & EQUIVALENT

DRY MEASUREMENTS CONVERSION CHART

3 TEASPOONS = 1 TABLESPOON = 1/16 CUP

6 TEASPOONS = 2 TABLESPOONS = 1/8 CUP

12 TEASPOONS = 4 TABLESPOONS = 1/4 CUP

24 TEASPOONS = 8 TABLESPOONS = 1/2 CUP

36 TEASPOONS = 12 TABLESPOONS = 3/4 CUP

48 TEASPOONS = 16 TABLESPOONS = 1 CUP

METRIC TO US COOKING CONVERSIONS

OVEN TEMPERATURE

120°C = 250° F

160°C = 320° F

180°C = 350° F

205°C = 400° F

220°C = 425° F

OVEN TEMPERATURE

8 FLUID OUNCES = 1 CUP = 1/2 PINT = 1/4 QUART

16 FLUID OUNCES = 2 CUPS = 1 PINT = 1/2 QUART

32 FLUID OUNCES = 4 CUPS = 2 PINTS = 1 QUART = 1/4 GALLON

128 FLUID OUNCES = 16 CUPS = 8 PINTS = 4 QUARTS = 1 GALLON

BAKING IN GRAMS

1 CUP FLOUR = 140 GRAMS

1 CUP SUGAR = 150 GRAMS

1 CUP POWDERED SUGAR = 160 GRAMS

1 CUP HEAVY CREAM = 235 GRAMS

VOLUME

1 MILLILITER = 1/5 TEASPOON

5 ML = 1 TEASPOON

15 ML = 1 TABLESPOON

240 ML = 1 CUP OR 8 FLUID OUNCES

1 LITER = 34 FL. OUNCES

WEIGHT

1 GRAM = .035 OUNCES

100 GRAMS = 3.5 OUNCES

500 GRAMS = 1.1 POUNDS

1 KILOGRAM = 35 OUNCES

US TO METRIC COOKING CONVERSIONS

1/5 TSP = 1 ML
1 TSP = 5 ML
1 TBSP = 15 ML
1 FL OUNCE = 30 ML
1 CUP = 237 ML
1 PINT (2 CUPS) = 473 ML
1 QUART (4 CUPS) = .95 LITER
1 GALLON (16 CUPS) = 3.8 LITERS
1 OZ = 28 GRAMS
1 POUND = 454 GRAMS

BUTTER

1 CUP BUTTER = 2 STICKS = 8 OUNCES = 230 GRAMS = 8 TABLESPOONS

BUTTER

1 CUP = 8 FLUID OUNCES
1 CUP = 16 TABLESPOONS
1 CUP = 48 TEASPOONS
1 CUP = 1/2 PINT
1 CUP = 1/4 QUART
1 CUP = 1/16 GALLON
1 CUP = 240 ML

BAKING PAN CONVERSIONS

1 CUP ALL-PURPOSE FLOUR = 4.5 OZ
1 CUP ROLLED OATS = 3 OZ 1 LARGE EGG = 1.7 OZ
1 CUP BUTTER = 8 OZ
1 CUP MILK = 8 OZ
1 CUP HEAVY CREAM = 8.4 OZ
1 CUP GRANULATED SUGAR = 7.1 OZ
1 CUP PACKED BROWN SUGAR = 7.75 OZ
1 CUP VEGETABLE OIL = 7.7 OZ
1 CUP UNSIFTED POWDERED SUGAR = 4.4 OZ

BAKING PAN CONVERSIONS

9-INCH ROUND CAKE PAN = 12 CUPS
10-INCH TUBE PAN = 16 CUPS
11-INCH BUNDT PAN = 12 CUPS
9-INCH SPRINGFORM PAN = 10 CUPS
9 X 5 INCH LOAF PAN = 8 CUPS
9-INCH SQUARE PAN = 8 CUPS

How to Reduce Food Waste

Plan Meals: Create a weekly meal plan and shopping list.

Store Food Properly: Use airtight containers and maintain the right temperature.

FIFO Rule: Consume older items before newer ones.

Portion Control: Serve smaller portions to avoid leftovers.

Use Leftovers: Repurpose or freeze them.

Understand Expiry Dates: Many foods are safe past these dates.

Composting: Start a compost bin for food scraps.

Donate: Share surplus non-perishables with food banks.

Shop Mindfully: Buy in bulk, choose minimal packaging.

Batch Cooking: Prep and freeze meals for later.

Preserve Foods: Learn canning, pickling, and drying.

Spread Awareness: Educate and inspire others.

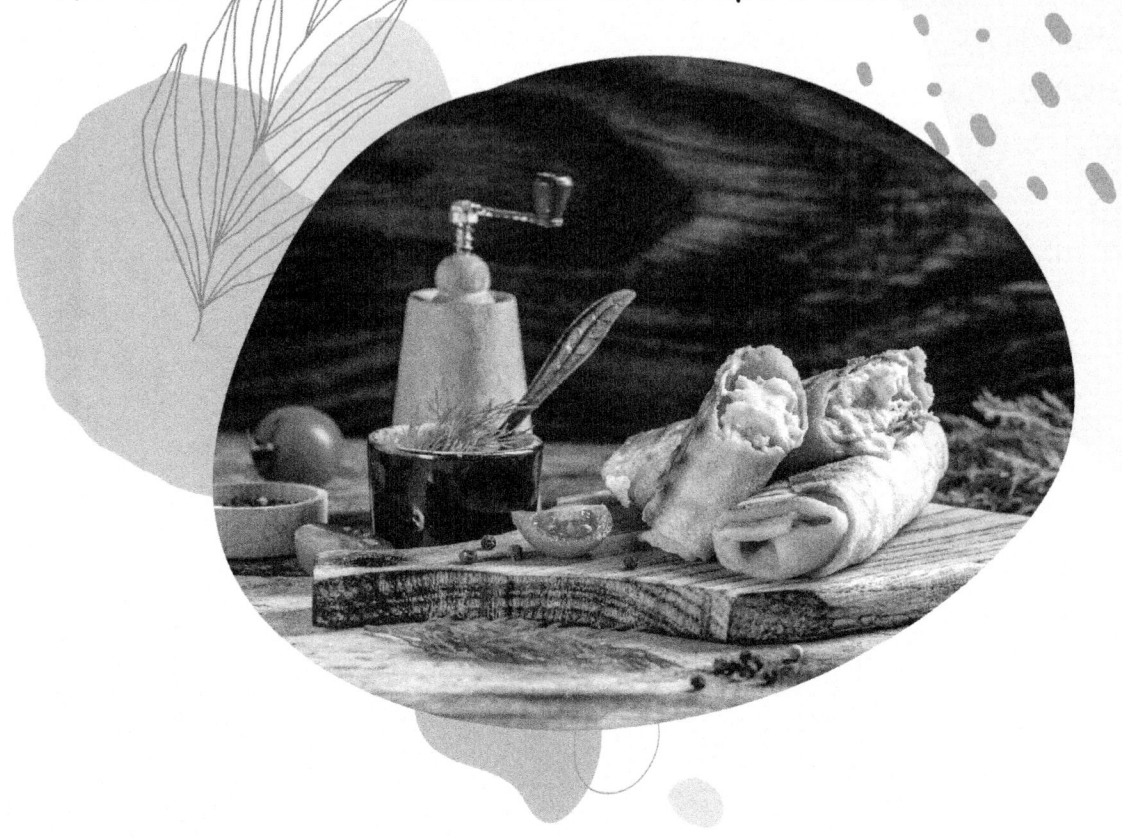

Recipe

From the kicthen of ....

Serves .... Prep time .... Cook time ....

☐ Difficulty ☐ Easy ☐ Medium ☐ Hard

Ingredient

Directions

Air Fryer Cookbook

APPENDIX : RECIPES INDEX

A

All-in-one Breakfast Toast 19
American Biscuits 21
Asian Five-spice Wings 24
Artichoke Samosas 28
Aubergine Parmigiana 36
Artichoke Pasta 38
Asian Glazed Meatballs 49
Asiago Broccoli 62
Almond-crusted Zucchini Fries 69
Asian-style Flank Steak 76
Annie's Chocolate Chunk Hazelnut Cookies 97
Apple Dumplings 97

B

Balsamic Marinated Rib Eye Steak With Balsamic Fried Cipollini Onions 77
Baked Eggs With Bacon-tomato Sauce 13
Breakfast Chimichangas 13
Buttermilk Biscuits 15
Beet Chips 25
Black-olive Poppers 26
Buffalo Bites 26
Buffalo Wings 27
Baba Ghanouj 29
Bbq Soy Curls 33
Butternut Squash Fries 33
Bagel Pizza 34
Broccoli Cheese 37
Black Bean Veggie Burgers 41
Best-ever Roast Beef Sandwiches 49
Beer-breaded Halibut Fish Tacos 53
Buttered Swordfish Steaks 54
Basil Crab Cakes With Fresh Salad 55

Basil Mushroom & Shrimp Spaghetti 56
Bbq Fried Oysters 57
Black Cod With Grapes, Fennel, Pecans, And Kale 59
Balsamic Beet Chips 62
Buttery Stuffed Tomatoes 65
Butternut Medallions With Honey Butter And Sage 67
Baked Shishito Peppers 70
Blackberry Bbq Glazed Country-style Ribs 73
Balsamic London Broil 74
Berbere Beef Steaks 75
Boneless Ribeye Steaks 75
Beef Brazilian Empanadas 78
Buttery Chicken Legs 85
Baked Apple 95
Black And Blue Clafoutis 96

C

Canadian Bacon & Cheese Sandwich 17
Cheddar & Egg Scramble 17
Crustless Broccoli, Roasted Pepper, And Fontina Quiche 19
Corn Dog Bites 23
Chicken Shawarma Bites 24
Cholula Avocado Fries 24
Chinese-style Potstickers 25
Cocktail Beef Bites 25
Classic Potato Chips 26
Cauliflower "tater" Tots 27
Charred Shishito Peppers 28
Cheddar Stuffed Pepper 28
Cayenne-spiced Roasted Pecans 30
Cheese, Tomato & Pesto Crustless Quiches 33
Courgette Meatballs 35
Camembert & Soldiers 36

Crispy Potato Peels 38
Chicken Apple Brie Melt 43
Chicken Spiedies 45
Chicken Saltimbocca Sandwiches 46
Chicken Gyros 47
Chili Cheese Dogs 48
Cajun Flounder Fillets 52
Caribbean Skewers 52
Coconut Jerk Shrimp 58
Californian Tilapia 60
Cheese Sage Cauliflower 64
Caraway Seed Pretzel Sticks 69
Corn On The Cob 70
Citrus Pork Lettuce Wraps 73
Crispy Pork Escalopes 75
Cinnamon-stick Kofta Skewers 76
Carne Asada Recipes 78
Carne Asada 79
Cajun Pork Loin Chops 80
Chipotle Pork Meatballs 80
Cal-mex Chimichangas 81
Chicken Strips 83
Chicken Chunks 85
Crunchy Chicken Strips 85
Chicken Flautas 86
Coconut Chicken With Apricot-ginger Sauce 86
Chicken Cordon Bleu 87
Cajun Fried Chicken 88
Chicago-style Turkey Meatballs 88
Cal-mex Turkey Patties 89
Chicken Flatbread Pizza With Spinach 89
Creole Chicken Drumettes 89
Chicken Cordon Bleu Patties 90
Crispy Chicken Parmesan 90
Caramel Apple Crumble 92
Chewy Coconut Cake 93
Cinnamon Canned Biscuit Donuts 95
Carrot-oat Cake Muffins 98
Coconut Macaroons 98

Chocolate Macaroons 99

D
Dijon Thyme Burgers 43
Dilly Red Snapper 57

E
Easy Caprese Flatbread 14
Egg & Bacon Pockets 15
Eggless Mung Bean Tart 16
Effortless Toffee Zucchini Bread 18
Egg And Sausage Crescent Rolls 20
Eggplant Parmesan Subs 47
Egg Stuffed Pork Meatballs 77

F
Favorite Blueberry Muffins 12
Feta & Shrimp Pita 53
Five-spice Roasted Sweet Potatoes 66
Fried Eggplant Balls 66
Fried Eggplant Slices 70
French-style Steak Salad 81
Farmer's Fried Chicken 84
Fast Brownies 95
Fried Twinkies 98

G
Garlic And Dill Salmon 54
Greek-inspired Ratatouille 67
Gorgonzola Stuffed Mushrooms 69
Glazed Meatloaf 74
Garlic-buttered Rib Eye Steak 80
Garlic Chicken 83
Granny Pesto Chicken Caprese 84
Gruyère Asparagus & Chicken Quiche 88
Glazed Cherry Turnovers 96

H
Ham & Cheese Sandwiches 14
Herby Parmesan Pita 17
Ham And Cheddar Gritters 18
Huevos Rancheros 20

Healthy Granola 21
Hot Garlic Kale Chips 29
Halibut With Coleslaw 57
Herb-rubbed Salmon With Avocado 59
Hot Calamari Rings 60
Hush Puppies 63
Honey-roasted Parsnips 64
Homemade Pork Gyoza 79
Harissa Chicken Wings 83
Honey-roasted Mixed Nuts 94

I

Indian Cauliflower Tikka Bites 23
Individual Pizzas 30
Inside Out Cheeseburgers 40
Inside-out Cheeseburgers 42
Irresistible Cheesy Chicken Sticks 87

L

Lemon Monkey Bread 12
Lime Bay Scallops 52
Lemon & Herb Crusted Salmon 54
Lime Flaming Halibut 60

M

Meaty Omelet 14
Mascarpone Iced Cinnamon Rolls 16
Mini Quiche 34
Mexican Cheeseburgers 40
Maple-crusted Salmon 51
Mahi-mahi "burrito" Fillets 55
Malaysian Shrimp With Sambal Mayo 56
Mahi Mahi With Cilantro-chili Butter 58
Mashed Sweet Potato Tots 63
Moroccan Cauliflower 68
Mango-chocolate Custard 92
Mixed Berry Pie 93
Molten Chocolate Almond Cakes 94
Mixed Berry Hand Pies 99

O

Orange Zingy Cauliflower 34

P

Potato Gratin 32
Paneer Tikka 35
Parmesan Truffle Oil Fries 37
Provolone Stuffed Meatballs 41
Perfect Burgers 44
Pecan-orange Crusted Striped Bass 51

R

Roast Cauliflower & Broccoli 32
Ratatouille 35
Reuben Sandwiches 48
Roasted Brussels Sprouts With Bacon 62

S

Sweet Potato Taquitos 32
Spicy Spanish Potatoes 33
Spinach And Egg Air Fryer Breakfast Muffins 37
Salmon Burgers 42
Sausage And Pepper Subs 45
Speedy Baked Caprese With Avocado 68
Street Corn 68
Stuffed Onions 71

T

Tomato And Herb Tofu 38
Turkey Burgers 44
Tuna Platter 65
Turkish Mutabal (eggplant Dip) 71

V

Vegan Fried Ravioli 36
Veggie Bakes 37

W

White Bean Veggie Burgers 46

Z

Za'atar Bell Peppers 64

Printed in Great Britain
by Amazon